Understanding Multiple Chemical Sensitivity

Understanding Multiple Chemical Sensitivity

Causes, Effects, Personal Experiences and Resources

ELS VALKENBURG

Foreword by KIM SCHOPPINK

McFarland & Company, Inc., Publishers
Jefferson, North Carolina, and London

Originally published as *Als chemische stoffen en geuren je ziek maken: Een naslagwerk over de onbegrepen milieuziekte MCS* (When Chemical Substances and Scents Make You Ill: A Reference Book about the Misunderstood Environmental Illness MCS) in the Netherlands in 2007 by Uitgeverij Schors, Amsterdam.

The information in this book is provided for educational purposes only. It is not intended as a substitute for medical treatment. The procedures, ideas and therapies described in the book should be discussed with a medical professional. The listing of specific products or methods does not constitute an endorsement of those products or methods. Because multiple chemical sensitivity varies considerably among individuals, it is each person's responsibility to make his or her own choices based upon personal research, testing of all materials, and professional medical advice.

The author and publishers of this book disclaim any liability arising directly or indirectly from the research and ideas presented in this book.— Els Valkenburg; translated by Jan P. Huisman.

ISBN 0-7864-4443-4
softcover : 50# alkaline paper ∞

LIBRARY OF CONGRESS CATALOGUING DATA ARE AVAILABLE

British Library cataloguing data are available

On the cover: The author wears an organic cotton mask (photograph by Ruurd Valkenburg); Labware photograph ©2010 Shutterstock

Manufactured in the United States of America

McFarland & Company, Inc., Publishers
Box 611, Jefferson, North Carolina 28640
www.mcfarlandpub.com

To all present and future MCS patients,
their partners, families, friends, doctors and relatives.
May this book contribute to increased understanding
and sympathy for the situation of the MCS patient,
so the love and care they need will not be denied.

Table of Contents

Acknowledgments

Thanks to all people, locally and globally, who spontaneously and unconditionally provided assistance with this book. Without them it would not have been produced in such a fantastic manner! Special thanks are due to Kim Schoppink of Greenpeace, who contributed the foreword.

Foreword by Kim Schoppink

More than one hundred thousand chemical substances are on the European* market. The majority of these are used in consumer products, many of which we use every day. We know of only three thousand of these chemicals and what effects they have on our environment and our health. This means it's possible that the products we use every day are not as safe as we think. Moreover, all chemicals eventually end up in the environment — pollution is caused when they are produced, and they leak from products during use and are released when products lie on the trash heap or are burned.

Countless chemical substances float around in our environment and in our bodies. We don't know what the individual effects of those substances are, not to mention the effects they have in combination. Greenpeace argues that chemicals should be allowed on the market only when their safety has been proven: prevention is better than cure. Greenpeace has been taking action towards a ban on toxic chemicals for years. We run campaigns against unsafe substances in cosmetics, athletic shoes and electronics. We also ring the alarm bell over the use of PVC and poisonous substances in ship paint. And we protest at the gates of the producers of these toxic chemicals. Some companies respond appropriately and replace chemicals, but others wait until legislation forces them to change.

With the new chemical legislation REACH, which was ratified in December 2006, Europe took a first step in the right direction. But much more needs to happen to protect our environment and ourselves against toxic chemicals. REACH will research the effects upon the environment and humans of a mere few thousand substances, but the effects of most substances we use will remain unknown. What's more, barely any attention will be paid to what happens when these chemical substances come together in nature or in our bodies. About these chemical cocktails we still know awfully little. It is possible this is a factor in Multiple Chemical Sensitivity as discussed in this book. Conclusive medical-scientific evidence for this is still lacking. Greenpeace argues that much more research ought to be done on the effects of chemical substances on our health and also on nature. There are scientific reports about the effects of dangerous chemicals on animals high up in the food chain, because they contain the high-

---

All industrialized nations are facing this same issue with chemical substances being released onto markets untested.

1

est concentrations. Even in the North Pole polar bears, whales, seals and humans are exposed to PCBs, dioxins, bromine-containing fire retardants, pesticides and other toxic substances. The harmful effects are becoming ever clearer. Early in 1998 Norwegian researchers discovered young polar bears with both male and female genitalia. In all likelihood there are many more animals getting sick from harmful chemicals.

Greenpeace demands an end to this gigantic experiment. Rather than being banned only after years of use have demonstrated their harmful effects, chemical substances should be regulated according to a principle of precaution: before a chemical is brought onto the market it must have been proven to be harmless. We will continue to strive for a toxin-free world.

Kim Schoppink
Greenpeace Netherlands, Amsterdam
Toxics Campaign Leader
www.greenpeace.nl

Preface

Dear reader,

You are about to learn more about an environmental illness which has been identified since the 1950s: Multiple Chemical Sensitivity (MCS).

People who suffer from this condition become ill from various (synthetic) chemical substances and/or scents and can barely lead a normal life, because these substances are almost everywhere. MCS is an invisible and often misunderstood condition that has driven many people into social isolation.

Increasing pollution harms the natural world (flora and fauna). The consequences — such as global warming — can be serious and in some cases disastrous. By now we know that many illnesses are caused by the environment we live in — almost 24 percent of all diseases, according to the World Health Organization (WHO). A report compiled by WHO (www.who.int/mediacentre/news/releases/2006/pr32/en/index.html) calls special attention to the two kinds of respiratory problems caused by indoor and outdoor environments.

Despite the many wake-up calls over the past years, it seems we prefer to keep sleeping. It would be naïve to think we humans could emerge from this merry-go-round unscathed, and that there will be no consequences for our DNA and the development of our children, given the daily use of an enormous amount of synthetic substances which have been shown to damage our living environment.

I had certainly hoped to start my book on a happier note, because I myself like to view everything optimistically, but I can't spin it any other way: we're facing a serious and growing health problem. I too never knew or wanted to know of the dangers in the chemicals and diverse chemical cocktails to which we are exposed every day — not for a second did I pause and consider that what I used, ate, drank and breathed was accumulating to the degree that the "bucket" eventually overflowed and there was no turning back. Not everyone's health will develop the same way as mine, as others may well have a better genetic profile or have less damaging circumstances in their life. Some will be spared this fate or experience it to a lesser degree. Knowing that exposure to chemical substances can cause genetic changes even in the womb should prompt humans to start making different choices. Mother Nature still has a lot of good and healthy things to offer.

Els Valkenburg

Introduction

Given the steady increase in the number of chemical sensitivities and allergies among adults and children, this book comes none too soon. This introduction outlines the reasons, motivations and goals of this book, and provides relevant comments from the author.

The Reasons

This book was written for the simple reason that worldwide, there is still not enough satisfactory information about MCS. Due to the lack of information and therefore the lack of relevant knowledge, MCS patients are often subject to ignorance and grave misunderstanding.

Most people are barely able to conceive of the fact that chemical substances and scents (even in small doses) can cause illness and lead to various, sometimes serious symptoms. Many people are presumed to suffer from MCS without themselves realizing that MCS causes their symptoms. They don't realize that their headaches or skin rashes might be caused by laundry detergent, a scented candle, the air freshener, a traffic jam, or even the office printer.

Many people consult their general practitioner for all kinds of complaints, both concrete and vague, such as respiratory problems, exhaustion, skin conditions, (chronic) infections, and so on, without finding effective help or a cure. The mainstream medical establishment often knows very little about chemical sensitivity.* Doctors and therapists have not been trained to look for or understand MCS and as a result this causation is rarely diagnosed. In order to connect the symptoms to MCS it is necessary to learn about the living environment and the home and work conditions of the patient. This takes more time than most doctors have available. Much improvement can be made in this regard.

The lives of MCS patients often are turned entirely upside down due to lack of thorough information on their condition. Some might even be forced to hermetically seal themselves from everyone in their surroundings who is unwilling or unable to adjust to the needs of the MCS patient. Accurate infor-

---

*Other than environmental health specialists, who are specifically trained to diagnose MCS (see entry 15 on page 18).

mation regarding the patient's health problems is often discovered far too late, allowing the situation to worsen over long periods of time as the patient is continuously exposed to various chemicals. In time the patient is unable to function in an environment where certain synthetic substances are present. For these people, participating in society in a normal way becomes impossible. This is a painful and sorry circumstance one wishes upon nobody, but especially not children!

Anyone can develop MCS, young or old. Almost every MCS patient will encounter a lack of sympathy, no matter how he tries to inform everyone in his immediate surroundings. A book such as this can help inform one's neighbors and loved ones in an independent and emotionally neutral way. Experience has shown that this improves understanding of the MCS patient's situation.

The Motivation

When, after many years, an MCS patient finally figures out what is going on, the thought often arises: "If only I had known sooner, I could have undertaken measures to prevent the condition from worsening." This thought provided the impulse to inform others on the subject of Multiple Chemical Sensitivity.

The website www.the-abc-of-mcs.com was one first big step towards creating awareness of MCS and educating patients, doctors, therapists, students and all other visitors to the website. This book is an inevitable and long overdue follow-up. MCS may be a largely unknown condition in most countries, but it constitutes a real and present problem nonetheless. A lot more people than one might not think of falling ill from their own perfume or cleaning detergents; it is high time for thorough worldwide public information on the matter.

The Goal

The author hopes this book will allow MCS patients and their partners, families and friends to improve their situation and their relationships (family, business, friendly) using the information presented here.

This book attempts to reach a large audience worldwide and thereby increase awareness and acceptance of MCS. Hopefully it will stimulate students, doctors and scientists to direct their attention towards MCS, with the aid of the scientific research presented in *Part I*. Such scientific engagement would bring general recognition of MCS by the medical community one step closer. Furthermore, this book aims to create an increased consciousness regarding the use of everyday products, including both foodstuffs and other consumer goods. Many people are quite trusting in this regard; rarely do we consider that countless products are made using synthetic substances. Even when they do not exceed legally permitted standards, such substances can still harm us and our children. We fail to realize that the vast majority of these synthetic substances have not undergone testing and that we do not know what long-term consequences these substances have for us and the environment. The possible dangers hidden in combinations of everyday synthetic substances (the so-called chemical cocktail) are also unknown or barely known, as Kim Schoppink points out in the foreword.

About This Book

This book is a report of the scientific aspects of the disease itself (see *Part I: What Is MCS?*) and a journal of personal experiences and an ethnography of life with MCS (see *Part II: The Personal Situation* and *Part III: The Voices of Others*). It contains tips, advice and information in several fields, and important addresses and links for the MCS patient (see *Part IV: The ABCs of MCS, Part V: Films, Books and Other Resources, Part VI: Further Resources*). In conclusion, *Part VII: Providing Information to Others*, is a guide that may help to inform others.

Comments

• The author does not intend this book to give the impression that all natural chemical substances are safe and only synthetic products are harmful to human beings. When it comes to chemical substances on Earth, such simplifications cannot be made.

• The author also is in no way intending to incite unrest or panic, or to assert that all chemical or synthetic substances are by definition harmful to everyone. After all, we all benefit from some scientific progress, such as the discovery of new and ever-improving medicines for AIDS, cancer, multiple sclerosis and, in time, perhaps for MCS!

• Some MCS patients become isolated. This does not mean, however, that isolation is the prognosis for everyone. There are very many people with chemical sensitivities who nevertheless are able to continue leading a normal life, because they were able to adjust and thereby improve their situation. The author hopes the information in this book will demonstrate that in the event of chemical sensitivity one must be extremely careful with daily and possible future exposures.

• Should you like to offer a response or comment on this book, please e-mail valkenburg@het-abc-van-mcs.nl.

PART I
What Is MCS?

1

MCS: General

1. What is MCS?

MCS stands for multiple chemical sensitivity and is also known as: CS (chemical sensitivity), CI (chemical injury), EI (environmental illness), TILT (toxicant-induced loss of tolerance), twentieth-century illness and IEI (idiopathic environmental intolerance). MCS is the most common term for this condition, and is used around the world.

People who suffer from this condition fall ill from diverse synthetic chemical substances and/or scents and, because these substances are found almost everywhere, are barely able to lead a normal life. MCS patients become ill from very low doses of chemical substances, to which a healthy person displays no noticeable reaction at all.

2. What are the causes of MCS?

There are many possible causes of MCS. At this time the best-known causes are:

• *long-term exposure* (years) to a "cocktail" of diverse, often low doses of chemical substances.

• *one-time exposure* to a high dose of a chemical substance, such as formaldehyde, solvents, insecticides, pesticides, toluene, anesthetic fluids and other chemical substances.

"Exposure" means inhalation, consumption, or otherwise coming into contact with chemical substances (such as via the skin).

3. What exactly are chemical substances?

In order to understand what is meant by "chemical substances," we must first ask ourselves what chemistry is. Chemistry is the science of the elements.

Chemistry plays an important role on earth. Life is actually all just chemistry and consists in large part of natural chemical substances and processes that allow for life and continued existence on Earth. Every being plays host to all kinds of natural chemical processes in all vital parts of the body. Composition, decomposition and the circulation of matter in the body are all chemical processes.

With the necessary knowledge of chemistry all kinds of substances can be produced, including substances that do not occur in nature. Raw materials from nature are used as the basis for synthetic products, of which plastic is a good example. Plastic is made using natural crude oil as primary product, and the final product is termed a "synthetic" product. The term "synthetic" indicates that a substance does not naturally occur and thus must be a fabricated product. Using chemical processes one can combine substances to create new ones, or one can separate substances. The purification of water (meaning the removal of harmful substances from water) is also a good example of such a chemical process. In everyday life we encounter both natural and synthetic chemical substances. Both can be very toxic (poisonous), particularly when used incorrectly or when one is exposed to a higher dose than is safe or permitted.

In this book, when "chemical substances" are mentioned, this should be taken to mean the "synthetic substances," unless the text expressly refers to natural substances.

4. Why are MCS patients sometimes called "canaries" or "yellow canaries"?

MCS patients are sometimes called canaries, because MCS patients can function as early warning signals. Early miners would take canaries down into the mine shafts because canaries fell from their perches rather quickly when carbon monoxide or other dangerous gases arose. Miners made sure they got out as soon as this happened. MCS patients are thus actually the canaries of this day and age, since they become ill from chemical substances in low doses, especially synthetic chemical substances, from which others do not (yet) get sick. They therefore also function as an alarm bell, although this bell is not heard as it should be.

5. Can anyone develop MCS?

Whether or not someone falls ill from chemical substances is mainly dependent on individual genetic predisposition and other factors (besides the fact that chemical substances can themselves cause genetic defects and MCS). Consider the fact that some people smoke heavily for their whole lives without suffering any health problems while others with the same unhealthy habit develop lung cancer and perish. Among the human population exists an enormous variation regarding genes and their mutations — among enzymes, for example, which break down substances foreign to the body. The same holds true for MCS patients.

As a result of this difference there will always be people who react with greater sensitivity to chemical substances than does the "average" human being. It is impossible to predict in advance who will develop MCS, because the condition is also dependent on what substances and situations a person encounters during his life. Everyone could thus develop it. MCS is a typical environmental illness of this day and age.

6. What are the most common signs and symptoms of MCS?

MCS patients react very differently after exposure to a substance that is harmful for them. For this reason the list of signs and symptoms is rather long, but this list does not suggest that all

MCS patients have experienced these symptoms or that MCS patients display all of them at the same time.

MCS is a multi-system disease, meaning that several organ systems are affected. (See *entry 24* for a definition of MCS.) This is the reason for the variation in symptoms.

- auto-immune system deficiencies
- blackouts
- brain fog
- breathing and respiratory problems
- cardiac arrhythmia
- chronic fatigue
- depression
- disorientation
- dizziness
- ear, nose, throat and sinus problems
- flu-like symptoms
- (food) allergies and intolerance
- general malaise — lethargy and weakness
- headaches
- inability to concentrate
- infections
- joint and muscle pain
- lung problems
- problems with short-term memory
- seizures
- sensitivity to electromagnetic fields
- skin diseases
- stomach and/or intestinal problems
- symptoms of poisoning (shivering, nausea, etc.)

7. Which substances can elicit a reaction?

An MCS patient reacts to all sorts of everyday chemical substances. Often it begins with a sensitivity to perfume, other scents or cigarette smoke. At this stage MCS is usually not recognized and no preventative measures towards avoiding chemical substances are taken. As a result new substances keep adding to the list of those to which the patient reacts — a clear characteristic of MCS.

Minimal concentrations of substances for which consequences for healthy people have not yet been identified can cause reactions in MCS patients — sometimes serious reactions.

Examples of substances to which MCS patients can have reactions:

- Air fresheners
- All products containing perfume
- Care products: deodorant, soap, shampoo, creams, toothpaste, etc.
- Cigarette and cigar smoke
- Combustion gases from geysers, ovens or gas furnaces
- Dish and laundry detergents
- Exhaust fumes
- Glue, paint, patina, etc.
- Insecticides, pesticides, etc.
- Medicine
- New construction materials and furniture
- New floor covering
- New or recently dry-cleaned clothes
- Paper, ink, newspapers, books, magazines, printers, etc.
- Plastics, plasticizer, rubber, etc.
- Smog and fine particles
- Smoke from fireplaces, stoves or barbecues
- Synthetic additives in food and drink

8. Is MCS an allergy like hay fever or an allergy to cats?

No, MCS does not fall under the "classic" allergies and can not be ascertained or proven with standard allergy testing. Many MCS patients have developed, aside from the chemical sensitivity, various allergies and food intolerances. As of yet there is no clear relation between MCS and allergies, although this too is strongly dependent on how allergies are defined. See "What Is Going On?" and "Allergy and MCS" at: www.satori-5.co.uk/word_articles/mcs/engaging_with_mcs.html.

9. People didn't get always sick from perfume, so why do they do so now?

In the past perfumes were made using flower and herb extracts and natural animal musk. These were very expensive and only used at special occasions. Nowadays perfume is 95 percent petrochemical substances (chemicals extracted from petroleum) and is much less expensive than the original "rose water" of yore, thus its use has become an everyday occurrence. Modern perfume can consist of hundreds of separate ingredients, and not all of these are tested for their effects upon health. Some ingredients could be toxic at certain dosage levels. Yet many still don't believe this, as if perfume is still just innocent natural extracts.

10. Does MCS overlap with other similar conditions?

There is overlap with, among others, ME/CFS (myalgic encephalomyelitis/chronic fatigue syndrome), Gulf War syndrome, chronic toxic encephalopathy (CTE or psycho-organic syndrome) and fibromyalgia. These diseases, among others, involve the same symptoms as MCS, such as joint and muscle pain, fatigue, impaired vision, respiratory problems, headaches, depression, dizziness, irritable bowel syndrome, chemical sensitivity and problems with memory, sleep, skin and concentration.

Professor Malcolm Hooper has conducted extensive research into these overlaps and the possible causes of various conditions. This research is worthwhile reading, but is quite complicated and scientific and is therefore not easily accessible to everyone. Via the website "The ABC of MCS" you can access a video presentation on the subject (as well as the images used) by Professor Hooper. See www.the-abc-of-mcs.com under "Movies, etc."

11. Aren't chemical substances tested for safety?

At the moment some one hundred thousand chemicals are in use, of which the majority is processed into consumer products. We know the short- and long-term consequences upon humans and the environment for only a fraction of these substances. What you buy in the store is thus not necessarily safe. In December 2006 Europe took a step towards better regulation of chemicals on the market; hopefully more countries will follow soon.

This legislation, called REACH (Registration, Evaluation and Authorization of Chemicals), was officially enacted on 1 July 2007. The law ensures that for thirty thousand substances more information will be disseminated, although only about 40 percent of these chemical substances will be researched for potential health and environmental risks. The remaining chemicals will continue to be shrouded in uncertainty. There is also very little research being done regarding the effects of all these substances combined, the so-called chemical cocktail. You can find more information about REACH at these links: http://ec.europa.eu/environment/chem icals/reach/reach_intro.htm and www. chemicalspolicy.org/downloads/REA CHisHere220307.pdf.

12. Aren't low concentrations harmless to humans?

This is often assumed, because we have been raised with this line of thinking. Chemical substances are so pervasive in our lives and we have gotten so used to their daily presence that we are deluded into feeling safe. We assume that the things in stores are safe for everyone even though this has usually not been proven. *See previous question.*

In any case it is unknown what the long-term effects of chemical substances will have for all of humanity, aside from the fact that the majority of chemical substances stay on the market until the substance is proven to have caused harm — a reversal of the burden of proof. When a chemical is proven to be harmful it is often replaced with another chemical of which there is also no certainty regarding its effects upon a person's health. Most chemical substances have simply not been charted and tested, to say nothing of the unknown consequences of combinations of different substances.

We are only a few generations along since the explosive growth of the chemical industry in the early 1950s, which, incidentally, is when the first cases were recorded of people becoming ill from chemical substances in the environment. At the time Dr. Theron Randolph called it "environmental illness," a term still used today. Nevertheless the rapid growth of this industry continues and new products enter the market every day. Humans are sometimes called the modern-day guinea pigs, but of course without an objective control as is customary in most animal testing laboratories.

13. Is MCS officially recognized in the United States?

There is no general recognition of MCS in the medical establishment, because of a lack of consensus about whether or not it is a distinct medical condition. The confusion is caused by a lack of a conclusive medical-scientific explanation for MCS, although several possible causes and mechanisms have been proposed. See *entry 27.*

For this reason, the U.S. medical establishment and some government health departments have still not officially recognized MCS as a disease. But, we hope, this is just a matter of time. The good news is that MCS is already recognized as a potentially disabling condition by the U.S. Department of Housing and Urban Development (HUD) and the Social Security Administration (SSA). Several MCS patients have won benefits in workers compensation cases. The Americans with Disabilities Act (ADA) protects people with disabilities from discrimination, including MCS patients. The ADA does not have a list of medical conditions that constitute disabilities; it just has a general definition of when a person is functionally disabled or not. Cases are judged on an individual basis. As a result, some MCS patients will receive disability benefits under the ADA while others will not. Although several government departments and other organizations recognize the condition, MCS patients still are confronted with negative attitudes when they seek treatment and help from professionals. There remains a lot of work to be done in this regard.

The first important step is to get your condition diagnosed by an environmental health specialist (see *entry 15*). If you have been injured on the job, it is best to find an attorney who is experienced in chemical exposure cases and personal injury claims.

For more information about the recognition of MCS in the United States, visit the following websites (see *Part VI* for government addresses as well):

From the U.S. Department of Housing and Urban Development

(HUD) the following is an interesting read: "MCS Disorder and Environmental Illness As Handicaps": www.hud. gov/offices/adm/hudclips/lops/GME-0 009LOPS.pdf

The U.S. Department of Education wrote "Information Memorandum RSA-IM-02-04: Multiple Chemical Sensitivity": www.ed.gov/policy/speced/ guid/rsa/im/2002/im-02-04.pdf

Multiple Chemical Sensitivities — Facts, Fiction, Disability and the Law By Gail Sullivan Restivo of Chemically Sensitive Living (CSL): www.lectlaw. com/filesh/csl01.htm

More about the Americans with Disabilities Act (ADA) for people suffering with MCS.

Job Accommodation Network (JAN) has information about: "How to Determine Whether a Person Has a Disability under the Americans with Disabilities Act (ADA)" www.jan.wvu.edu/cor ner/vol02iss04.htm

For additional information regarding whether MCS is a disability, see the following letter: www.jan.wvu.edu/lette rs/EEOCLetter_MCS_Disability_July_ 96.doc

MCS Referral & Resources has a list of policies, court decisions and several organizations that recognize MCS: www.mcsrr.org/factsheets/mcsrecog. html and www.mcsrr.org/factsheets/ MCSrecogn.pdf

MCS America has lots of information on the current MCS situation.

For example, see its "Position Statement": http://mcs-america.org/MCSP ositionStatement.pdf

14. What about recognition in other countries?

In some countries there is greater acceptance of MCS and in some cases there is a partial recognition by the government. Although a general medical recognition of MCS as a disease exists nowhere, a diagnosis of MCS can be made in some countries.

CANADA

In Canada more progress has been made in the recognition of MCS than in most countries of the world. Canada took many measures to improve the lives of MCS patients and others who have environmentally induced respiratory problems, like asthma patients. See, for example, the brochure of the Canadian Lung Association: www.nb.lung. ca/pdf/NoScentsMakeSense.pdf

Just like the U.S., Canada has several clinical ecological centers to help diagnose and support people with environmental illnesses.

An important document from the Canadian Human Rights Commission about the recognition of MCS by the Canadian federal government and national bodies: www.chrc-ccdp.ca/pdf/envsensitivity_en.pdf or www.chrc-ccdp.ca/research_program_recherche/ese nsitivities_hypersensibilitee/toc_tdm-en.asp

See page 3 for their information about international recognition.

Canada also has an entirely scent-free city: Halifax! Canada takes all sorts of measures to make hospitals, office build-

ings and schools scent free. In the United States such measures are also taken at some universities and schools. For many links on this subject, go to www.the-abc-of-mcs.com, under "Perfume (free)."

DENMARK

The Danish Environmental Protection Agency published a very interesting and comprehensive report on the current situation regarding the recognition of MCS in Europe, Canada and the U.S. (In Denmark, MCS is called odor and chemical hypersensitivity.) For the English version of this document, go to: Environmental Project no. 988, 2005 http://www2.mst.dk/Udgiv/publicat ions/2005/87-7614-548-4/html/helep ubl_eng.htm

Or go to:

1. www.mst.dk
2. on the top left at "Udgivelser" go to "Rapporter" and then to "2005"
3. on the top right fill in the title project and number and year and click on "Søg."

GERMANY

Germany is the leader in Europe concerning the recognition and support of MCS patients. Germany has several environmental health centers, and in Germany it is possible to receive an MCS diagnosis based on the World Health Organization (WHO) classification of diseases ICD10-T78.4 (Allergy, unspecified). See www.who.int/occupati onal_health/publications/en/oehicd10.p df.

Although a diagnosis can nowadays

be made in Germany, this does not mean an MCS patient automatically gets official recognition or disability benefits. That depends on the personal situation, the medical file and the court decision.

15. How can you be diagnosed with MCS?

The best thing to do when you suspect you have MCS (of course, you will already have ruled out other possible causes for your ailments by seeing your general practitioner), is to seek help and eventually a diagnosis from an environmental health specialist/center or from a physician specializing in environmental medicine.

The American Academy of Environmental Medicine (AAEM) has many international members (physicians and other professionals) who are all specialists in environmental illnesses:

AAEM
6505 E. Central Avenue, #296
Wichita, KS 67206
Phone: (316) 684-5500

Go to www.aaemonline.org for more information and physicians' addresses.

Or ask for advice and help at one of the environmental health centers in the U.S.:

Center for Occupational and Environmental Medicine
7510 Northforest Drive
North Charleston, SC 29420
Phone: (843) 572-1600
http://coem.com

Environmental Health Center–Dallas
8345 Walnut Hill Lane, Suite 220

Dallas, TX 75231
Phone: (214) 368-4132
www.ehcd.com

Johnson Medical Associates
101 S. Coit Rd., Suite 317
Richardson, TX 75080
Phone: (972) 479-0400 or (800) 807-7555
www.johnsonmedicalassociates.com

Robbins' Environmental Medicine Center
420 West Hillsboro Blvd.
Deerfield Beach, FL 33441
Phone: (954) 421-1929 or (561) 395-3282
http://allergycenter.com

Also see *entry 298* for more (international) environmental health centers and a few websites from well-known physicians, or go to www.the-abc-of-mcs.com.

Here are some informational links to help you find a doctor:

American College of Occupational and Environmental Medicine
www.acoem.org

Doctors Treating MCS and/or CFS/FM Nationwide
http://mcs-america.org/doctorlist.pdf

Here are some informational links about other diagnosis protocols:

Biomarkers of MCS
www.mcsrr.org/resources/biomarkers.html

Defining Chemical Injury
Diagnostic Protocol by G. Heuser, et al.
www.iicph.org/docs/ipph_Defining_Chemical_Injury.htm

Environmentally Triggered Disorders
Dr. W. J. Rea, Environmental Health Center-Dallas
www.aehf.com/articles/A19.htm

Also see *entries 24* and *25* for the definition of MCS.

16. Are there mainstream doctors who take MCS seriously?

Fortunately, there are already some general practitioners and doctors who take MCS patients very seriously and cooperate in trying to improve their situation, but the majority of medical doctors have not been trained in environmental illnesses and often do not understand MCS very well. When visiting specialists within the mainstream medical establishment, many MCS patients are met with disbelief or the judgment that it's "all in your head," since these specialists cannot find a clear explanation for their symptoms using conventional diagnostic models.

The lack of support from physicians causes great stress to MCS patients, and when the MCS patient is prescribed conventional medicine to treat certain symptoms, the situation could even get worse in reaction to the medicine. Treatment with antidepressants — used because the doctor thinks the condition is psychosomatic — can cause other serious health problems, according to the experience of MCS patients and specific research (see *entry 21* about which therapies are found to be helpful).

Physicians who take MCS seriously and tend to be more helpful to the patient are occupational and environmental health specialists. Of course, it is always a good idea to inform your own mainstream doctor about MCS, especially if your doctor does not seem to know much about it. Some mainstream doctors really do care and are open to learning new things and gaining new insights, though so far they still seem in the minority.

17. How do you know you have MCS and not something else?

MCS is caused by exposure to chemical substances (either a single high-dose exposure or low-dose exposures over a long period of time; see *entry 2*). Often, due to the symptoms and the reactions to various (low dose) chemical substances, it is clear that MCS is at hand, especially when there is also an obvious cause. Of course, the other possible causes of the health situation must be ruled out, since cures exist for many other diseases and naturally the focus must be on those at first. So one ought to conduct all regular tests and studies (consult with your doctor) in order to rule out all other possible physical factors. Some symptoms characteristic of other conditions can resemble the symptoms of MCS but do not "officially" fall within them, such as asthmatic diseases (though people with asthma may have developed MCS on the side).

MCS patients have in general traversed the entire medical circuit and received from various specialists the comment "You are perfectly healthy," although they feel sick as can be. They often discover by themselves that they have begun reacting to certain chemical substances and that increasingly limits them in their freedom, so that they can't but keep looking for answers to their questions as to what is afflicting them. In their search, their own persistence oftentimes points them to MCS.

18. Do MCS patients also react to natural scents?

Yes, there are people who, as their condition develops, begin reacting to various natural scents. But as a rule MCS initially develops after exposure to chemical (synthetic) substances. Fortunately there are also MCS patients who can enjoy to the fullest a fragrant flower in the yard or use 100 percent natural (organic) scented soaps, shampoos and oils, without becoming ill. From their own natural scents and gases they usually do not get sick. *See next question.*

19. Can an MCS patient become ill from something which has no scent?

MCS is a sensitivity to chemical substances. After all, this disease is named multiple chemical sensitivity and not multiple *scent* sensitivity. A person can react to all sorts of scents, but this does not mean that if something does not smell, it won't make a person ill. Speaking of "sensitivity to scents" is thus a bit misleading and can cause misunderstanding and confusion, leading people to ask "Can't I even smell nice anymore?" even if those same people do understand the fact that you can be affected by chemical substances.

After all, everyone knows these substances can be dangerous or unhealthy. Most synthetic substances, such as perfume, body care products and dish and laundry detergents have a scent. We usually do not react to the scent but to the chemical substance that produces this scent. That is a big difference! There are many people who react to essential (or aromatic) oils, but who forget that there usually is nothing natural about these oils any more, meaning the scents are likely to be synthetic rather than natural. (These oils would be far too expensive if produced naturally.) Though there may be many differences among MCS patients, this disease is characterized mostly by the fact that people become ill from chemical or synthetic substances. True, other sensitivities exist as well. Still, this does not make us a group of people who are unable to enjoy natural scents.

2

MCS: Treatment and Strategies for Relief

20. What can you do about MCS?

According to several MCS doctors and scientists and MCS patients themselves, living in a chemical-free environment and thereby avoiding harmful substances is the most effective solution, difficult as this can be. There are supporting therapies that can provide relief, but these have not been proven to solve the problem because the cause is not addressed. *See the next question* for the results of a study among MCS patients regarding the most effective coping strategy. Also see *entries 22* and *23*.

21. Which treatment is found to be most helpful?

Research has been done among almost a thousand MCS patients into therapies and treatments that proved most effective. The results can be found online at the following website: www.eh ponline.org/members/2003/5936/5936. html. From this research it became apparent that MCS patients benefit most from a chemical-free living environment and the consequent avoidance of chemical substances. Prescribed medication was found to be least helpful.

Elements of treatment that scored over 75 percent and were thus considered most helpful are:

Chemical-free living space	94.8%
Chemical avoidance	94.5%
Relocation	86.6%
Air filter (to prevent exposure)	82.1%
Personal oxygen after exposure	78.4%
Charcoal mask	77.4%
Support groups	75.9%

In the study several therapies are mentioned, but these scored far lower than 75 percent.

22. How do you make a house as safe as possible?

Although all MCS patients react differently and must in large part "reinvent the wheel" by discovering which substances make them ill, you will find some general instructions and assistance below. For the severe MCS patient many adjustments are a bitter necessity, while for the "mild" MCS patient these tips are designed to prevent a worsening of the situation. Not all suggestions will be applicable to everyone in their current situation.

• You can make your house safe by taking out all unsafe substances (at least all those substances that make you sick), even if this means removing your recently laid new floor covering or your new cabinets. In general it can be said that all new things are unsafe for MCS patients, as new products give off all sorts of substances, a good example being formaldehyde.

• When furnishing your home, choose among natural, organic and MCS-safe materials as much as possible (see *entries 177* and *235*), or use secondhand materials that do not release harmful gases. When choosing secondhand materials, do make sure that smoke or perfume from previous owners has not already contaminated the product.

• It's preferable to gas out new materials in a well-ventilated space which you do not have to enter. Keep in mind that you can react to natural materials as well, especially if these are not organically produced and if — aside from MCS — you also have allergies or sensitivities to natural substances. Also keep in mind that the "green" label does not necessarily mean the product is nontoxic.

• Particularly when using paint or other materials on walls, ceilings and floors it's advisable to proceed very carefully (see *Part IV: The ABCs of MCS*). No MCS patient has exactly the same problems, so it is best not to adopt someone else's advice without considering whether it suits your own situation.

• Purchase a good air purifier, so you will breathe purified air inside your own home. To make air purifiers most effective, however, it is also necessary to remove the things that are making you ill. The air purifier itself also needs to be tested to see if you can tolerate it. Ask to bring a device home for a tryout. Realize that even a specifically "MCS-safe" air purifier must first be gassed out for a while and that you should run the device in another room for a period of time be-fore you test it or start using it. Giving your air purifier enough time to become safe for you is always preferable to not buying one. Take the time to scope out the options before buying an air purifier, since many do not work effectively due to their insufficient filter medium or because the housing is made from very unsuitable materials (see *entry 144*).

• In some cases, if you are living in an area with lots of air pollution or have neighbors who constantly set off your triggers, it's best to move to a safer residence or neighborhood. If after several adjustments and measures your house is still not safe for you (don't give up too quickly), moving is almost your only option — though it's not easy to find another MCS-safe house just like that. You risk jumping out of the frying pan and into the fire, since your new house and environment might contain other chemical substances that make you ill.

• Some people who are approaching desperation and are unable to live inside almost anywhere, choose to live in an RV or specifically designed MCS cabin in their own yard. See *Part VI* for several links concerning MCS housing.

• If you move into a newly (not ecologically) constructed home the problems are usually grave, because almost everything could cause problems: the walls, the heating system, the new kitchen cabinets, and so forth. The approach in this case is to ensure at least a single safe room and to live only in this room. Hopefully the walls, floors and so forth will become safe for you as soon as possible. Otherwise it is better to move to a temporary residence in an RV or something similar. Indeed, for new homes, it's advisable to place a quality air purifier in each room, running day and night until the fumes are mitigated. Do not remain in a place or room that makes you ill, for this could seriously deteriorate your situation.

• New appliances must first be gassed out for a long time. The gases that emanate from a new PC or TV, for example, can make you quite ill (among other reasons due to the bromine-containing fire retardant substances these devices often contain nowadays). Heat will cause a TV or PC to gas out more quickly, so it's good to let them run in another room, if necessary using a time switch. If you just leave the TV in a box up in the attic for a year before using it, you run the risk of still suffering from gases when the TV heats up. Also see *entry 191* for tips.

• If you recently changed or renewed something in your home and now you are experiencing symptoms, you should start by reversing these changes to see if the situation improves. For this reason it's best to never implement more than one change in your home at a time; the balance is somewhat fragile in this regard.

• Flowers and plants from garden centers and stores have often been sprayed with chemicals, so you should bar them from your home as much as possible if they recently came from the garden center. Letting plants first release chemical gases in another room is a good option. For websites about organic flowers, see *Part VI.*

• Newspapers and magazines are best left out of your home; use the Internet to read and research everything (assuming you do not react to your computer). Do not leave stacks of old paper or new

books and magazines in your safe room. If you do wish to keep a magazine in your living room, a reading box could be a good solution. Do keep in mind that when you open the reading box, gases could be released. For more information on how to build your own reading box, see an example at http://au.geo cities.com/dj_ludlow/mcs/readboxin tro.pdf. Or look for Cellophane Reading Bags at www.needs.com.

• Make sure the windows and doors are tightly sealed, so the smoke from your neighbor's barbeque grill or furnace, exhaust from traffic and smog cannot enter your home. Do ventilate your house during safe hours, because a space that is never ventilated quickly becomes unsafe due to the risk of mold! For taping gaps in your windows and doors, aluminum foil tape has proven very suitable, though of course not very useful for swiveling parts. See *entry 149.*

• Do not use chemical/synthetic cleaning detergents or air fresheners; these pollute the air in your home and can cause health problems. There are many other healthy alternatives. See *entries 174* and *184.*

• Ensure that your bedroom becomes a safe oasis within your home. Use organic sheets and bedding. See *entry 156.*

• Try to limit the amount of "electro smog" in your home. Many MCS patients are sensitive to radiation from cordless phones, screens and monitors, electricity from waterbeds, chairs, and the like, or will start to develop this sensitivity rapidly. See *entry 189.*

• Do not let people into your home who are not safe for you. Try as much as possible to inform them ahead of time, so they are willing and able to accommodate your situation. If they follow a thorough list of instructions you provide them and if they use the products you ask them to, home visits will once again be possible. (See *entry 225* for an example of a list of instructions.)

• You can also ask handymen, contractors and other visitors if they could arrive as perfume- and aftershave-free as possible. If somebody comes by often, you can give them safe products for washing (clothes and body), which reduces a large part of the harmfulness. Often people are willing to cooperate, especially when it costs them no money. Another option is to ask someone to put on a Tyvek coverall (see *entry 306* and *Part VI* for online vendors).

• Do not let visitors who are not safe for you (chemical- or scent-free) sit on your furniture; the fabric could absorb the perfume scents from their clothes. Protect your couch with Tyvek (available at stores that sell kite-making materials), or ask your visitors to sit on smooth (plastic) garden chairs which are easy to clean and put away.

• If a courier or deliveryman is standing in front of your door while smoking a cigarette, ask him to first put out the cigarette before you open the door. Often you can speak through the door. If an engine is still running right in front of your door, ask them to first turn it off. Perhaps you could hang a sign on your door with the words: "Please turn off engine, then ring bell" and point to it if you can't open the door. After all, it's a shame that such a short moment of exposure should allow harmful substances to enter your home, with negative consequences for you.

The idea is to make your home safe with a well-considered management strategy. Old materials, which might have caused problems when new, don't necessarily have to be torn from your house because in general they've long released all their gases. Try as much as possible to focus on the sources of your illness and do not in a frenzy start overhauling your entire house. (See *Part IV: The ABCs of MCS* for tips and suggestions).

23. How do you make your life safer in general?

• Consistently avoiding all chemical/synthetic substances and scents that make you sick usually quickly reduces symptoms. In some cases a temporary (social) isolation is necessary. You will start to discover that by making certain sacrifices you will be rewarded and will soon start to feel happier and better.

• It should go without saying that quitting smoking is an essential step. Secondhand smoke is also very harmful to your condition. After all, cigarette smoke contains over four thousand different chemicals that your body will have to process!

• Protect yourself from places and situations that are unsafe by immediately walking away or wearing an MCS mask, a half- or full-face respiratory mask, or by wearing a helmet with a portable air purifier. See *entry 274* for more information.

• Train yourself to be able to hold your breath for a while, should this be necessary.

• As much as possible, avoid going to shopping malls, crowded streets or other venues where people are wearing perfume or where people are smoking.

• Realize that harmful chemical substances are present in the air, in the water, in your food, clothing, care products, food supplements, and virtually everywhere. Find the sources of your negative physical reactions in all areas and adjust your life on as many levels as possible.

• Replace dish, laundry and cleaning detergents as much as possible with products that are made from 100 percent natural substances and organically produced; "perfume-free" does not necessarily imply that a laundry detergent does not contain synthetic substances! It may not have a scent, but it can still make you sick. It's a matter of figuring out which product seems to work for you. See *entries 174* and *184* for the various possibilities.

• Use only personal care products which are completely safe and tolerable for you. Here too you must find out which products you can tolerate. The safest tend to be all-natural and especially organic products, but if you react to natural substances and pure essential oils, then you must look hard to find out what is and isn't possible. See *entry 262* for more suggestions.

• Use chlorine- and perfume-free toilet paper (widely available in natural/organic products stores and some supermarkets) to spare the skin and perhaps place a chlorine filter on your shower: this prevents negative reactions to possible chlorine vapor while showering.

• Purify your water using a water purification system (visit www.the-abc-of-mcs.com under "Water & Oxygen" and *entry 312* for the possibilities), or drink mineral water. Tap water contains chemical substances and in all cases chlorine, since this is used to decontaminate the water. They may be legally permitted levels of chlorine, but these could still be aggravating the condition of an MCS patient.

• Eat organic foods as much as possible (at the very least avoid food with aromatic, color, taste and other synthetic additives). Fruits and vegetables in regular supermarkets were often contaminated with pesticides which could elicit a negative physical reaction in an MCS patient. Some areas have also a natural foods store where tasty and healthy food can be purchased. For meat eaters there are also organic butchers who sell healthy and organic meat. Just Google "organic meats" or ask your local health food store for possibilities or addresses. See *entry 248*.

• Avoid alcohol (ethanol), because alcohol is processed into poisonous acetaldehyde, a substance more poisonous and harmful than alcohol itself. The liver must subsequently break down this harmful substance, which is an extra burden upon the liver of a MCS patient, especially when this patient also has a defective cytochrome P450 liver enzyme (see *entry 27*).

• Avoid as much refined sugar as possible ("refined" meaning "produced at a refinery"). These sugar products are manufactured using chemical substances and processes, so choose natural, unrefined sugars. See *entry 293*.

• Try as much as possible to detoxify by relieving your body from breathing or otherwise consuming chemical substances, regularly using a (safe) sauna, exercising, drinking pure water, practicing Reiki, and using supplements and homeopathic products to support detoxification (preferably with the aid of an experienced therapist). In *Part IV: The ABCs of MCS* more information can be found about these various methods of detoxification. *See also next point.*

• Be careful using food supplements prescribed by a therapist who is not sufficiently knowledgeable about MCS and the problems engendered by an impaired detoxification process due to damaged detoxification paths in the liver, which often occurs with MCS patients (see *entry 27*). In consultation with your therapist, start by taking smaller than normal doses and slowly build up to a higher dose, to avoid a pile-up and poisonous reactions. The best way to take supplements is to get treated by an environmental health specialist.

• Stress can worsen your MCS symptoms due to the adrenalin boosts (internal triggers) which your body must process. Especially when the patient has a damaged detoxification system this could mean an added burden. Meditation and Reiki are quick methods to relax a stressed body and soul. See *entries 238* and *272.*

• If ink makes you sick, avoid opening mail without protection; write using a pencil instead of a pen or marker. Let recently printed documents and photographs gas out before you view them or use a gassed-out Ziploc bag. Do not read new books or magazines without protection if these make you sick, but place the book in a gassed-out big see-through plastic bag (perhaps with a

zipper) or use a reading box (see *entry 271*).

• Allow new clothes to gas out and repeatedly wash them before use. ("Normal" clothing is manufactured using many chemicals, such as pesticides in cotton, bleach, synthetic paints, chemicals in the production process and in the shipping containers, and so on. Of course, it's best not to wear clothes which were recently dry-cleaned, unless the dry cleaner is "green" and does not use harmful chemicals! Either way it is good to be very careful and to be well-informed as to whether you want to use this "green" alternative. "Green" does not necessarily mean safe for MCS patients. See *Part VI* for more information and addresses on this subject, as well as the following links: http://en.wikipedia.org/wiki/GreenEarth_Cleaning; www.naturalnews.com/023365.html; www.drycleaningstation.com

• Do not shine your shoes yourself but ask someone else to do it for you. If you must do it yourself, always make use of respiratory protection. Always allow recently shined shoes to gas out before wearing them (or use an alternative shoeshine product that is safe for you). Do not forget to also gas out new shoes for a long time, unless you have bought shoes made with natural or organic materials. See *entry 279.*

• If you are still working, it's a good idea to inform your boss and colleagues about MCS and try to cultivate understanding and respect for your situation, which won't be easy. Perhaps a move to a separate workspace is within the possibilities and you can place a portable air purifier there. You can also ask your colleagues not to enter your office if they are wearing perfume, and to contact you by telephone as much as possible. Do not forget to hang a sign on your door and perhaps protect yourself with a mask or helmet when walking through the building. In many situations you may have no choice but to find another work environment where your sensitivity is not such a great problem (which won't be many environments — working at home is one of the best options in this regard).

When you have made all the necessary adjustments and you are being supported by an environmental health specialist or any other doctor who can treat MCS (you probably have already started to feel better after a few months), it's important to shift your focus toward learning to accept life with MCS. (Certainly in this case all other medical causes of your condition should have already been ruled out through the established medical arena.) With this new attitude you will find in time that you reach inner acceptance and peace, and thereby avoid being stuck in a downward spiral. The disadvantage of denial is that you continue to expose yourself to all sorts of substances and risk becoming sensitive to even more substances.

See *Part IV: The ABCs of MCS* for tips and suggestions.

3

MCS: Scientific

I am myself not well grounded in science, but I wanted to compile a report of the current state of affairs, without meaning to give the impression that MCS is at this point thoroughly understood by the medical community.

If you want to dig deeper into the scientific findings described in this chapter, there are links and references for your convenience, so you can find the complete and original texts or more detailed information relevant to the issue at hand.

24. What is the definition of MCS?

The most commonly accepted definition of MCS was written by Mark Cullen, M.D., a professor of medicine and epidemiology at Yale University. In "Workers With Multiple Chemical Sensitivities," *Occupational Medicine* 2 (1987): 655–626, he writes, "Multiple chemical sensitivities is an acquired disorder characterized by recurrent symptoms, referable to multiple organ systems, occurring in response to demonstrable exposure to many chemically unrelated compounds at doses far below those established in the general population to cause harmful effects. No single widely accepted test of physiologic function can be shown to correlate with symptoms."

You may wish to visit some links

that discuss Cullen's definition: www.health.gov/environment/mcs/toc.htm and www.health.gov/environment/mcs/I.htm.

25. How can MCS be diagnosed?

In the literature references are often made to a number of clinical diagnostic criteria for establishing MCS (see sources below). They are:

1. The symptoms are reproducible by means of repeated chemical exposures.

2. The condition is chronic.

3. Low levels of exposure (lower than previously or commonly tolerated) result in manifestations of MCS.

4. Symptoms improve when the triggers are removed, but the problem itself remains.

5. Responses occur to multiple chemically unrelated substances.

6. Symptoms occur in multiple organ systems.

Also see next question.

SOURCES

J. R. Nethercott et al., "Multiple Chemical Sensitivities Syndrome: Toward a Working Case Definition," *Archives of Environmental Health* 1993; 48:19–26. www.ncbi.nlm.nih.gov/pubmed/8452395?dopt=Abstract.
L. Barta et al., "Multiple Chemical Sensitivity (MCS) : A 1999 Consensus," *Archives of Environ-*

mental Health 1999; 54(3):147–149. www.
elc.org.uk/pages/healthmcsdefinition.htm.

26. Which tests can be used to diagnose MCS?

Environmental health specialists can use a great number of research methods to ascertain the presence of MCS, partially due to the diversity among symptoms and partially because of the fact that the whole body is affected by MCS. The tests concern, among other things, blood and urine samples, allergy and skin tests, SPECT-scans, biopsies, and neuro-cognitive tests. Below you can find three websites which report extensively on the employed methods and the results of studies.

Biomarkers of MCS
www.mcsrr.org/resources/biomark
ers.html

Defining Chemical Injury
G. Heuser, P. Axelrod and S. Heuser
www.iicph.org/docs/ipph_Defining_
Chemical_Injury.htm

Environmentally Triggered Disorders
W. J. Rea, Environmental Health
Center-Dallas
www.aehf.com/articles/A19.htm

27. What is the medical explanation for the cause and mechanisms of MCS?

At this time (2009) there is no conclusive medical-scientific explanation for MCS and some controversy still exists over whether MCS is physical or psychosomatic (see also *entry 28*). The following are a few important findings and theories concerning the possible causes of MCS.

GENETICS

MCS may be partially related to genetic defects. A 2004 study demonstrated for the first time the genetic differences between people who suffer from MCS and those without such sensitivities. In 2007 another study resulted in the same findings regarding the correlation between certain genetic differences and the occurrence of MCS.

The 2004 study, titled "Case-control Study of Genotypes in Multiple Chemical Sensitivity: CYP2D6, NAT1, NAT2, PON1, PON2, and MTHFR," by McKeown-Eyssen et al., was published in the *International Journal of Epidemiology* and is available online: http://ije.oxfordjournals.org/cgi/reprint/dyh 251vl.

A seminar discussing these findings, "Genetic Differences Predict Multiple Chemical Sensitivity," can be found on the website of the group Protecting Our Health: www.protectingourhealth.org/newscience/immune/2004/2004-0715 mckeown-eyssenetal.htm. More information on McKeown-Eyssen's research can be found on the website of the University of Toronto's Faculty of Medicine: www.utoronto.ca/nutrisci/faculty/McKeown-Eyssen.

An interesting article by Angela Spivey entitled "Genes and Sensitivity" can be found in *Environmental Health Perspectives*, online at www.ehponline.org/docs/2005/113-3/forum.html#gene.

The 2007 study, "A Cross-Sectional Study of Self-Reported Chemical-

Related Sensitivity Is Associated with Gene Variants of Drug-metabolizing Enzymes," by Eckart Schnakenberg et al., was published in *Environmental Health* and can be read at www.ncbi. nlm.nih.gov/pubmed/17291352?dopt=A bstract.

IMMUNOLOGY

Dr. William Rea of the Environmental Health Clinic in Dallas, Texas, describes disturbances to the immune system as a result of exposure to chemical substances. He speaks of a "Total Body Overload," whereby the body is completely overwhelmed with chemical substances and unable to process them properly.

Dr. Rea's approach to treatment includes consistent programs of avoidance, neutralizing injections (for allergies/intolerances), detoxification therapies using a sauna, massages and exercise programs in controlled environments and vitamins and minerals.

An interview with Dr. Rea can be found at www.johnleemd.com/store/ env_illness.html, entitled "Environmental Illness: Could Chemical Overload Be the Cause of Your Illness?" More information is available in many medical articles on environmental aspects of health and disease, on the American Environmental Health Foundation (AEHF) website, www.aehf.com/articles/Med Artl.html.

Dr. Rea is the founder of the AEHF and director of the Environmental Health Clinic in Dallas, Texas. You can view an overview of his professional career at www.ehcd.com/center/profession albios.html.

LIMBIC SENSITIVITY— HYPOTHALAMUS DISORDER

Another theory regarding the possible cause of MCS involves a disorder in the hypothalamus, a member of the limbic system. The hypothalamus is a segment of the diencephalon which lies directly below the thalamus. The hypothalamus is a control center for the functioning of the pituitary gland and autonomic nervous system. The limbic system has a strong connection to the segment of our brain that controls our ability to smell and our nasal organ. A number of researchers suggest that the brain and particularly the limbic system can become hypersensitive to small amounts of chemicals. One of the functions of the limbic system is the management of moods and the functions of the central nervous system. This would explain why the symptoms of MCS also affect one's mood.

Animal testing has also demonstrated that animals exposed once to a high dose of chemicals or to a low dose of chemicals over a long period of time became hypersensitive such that additional exposures to chemicals began to affect the electrical activity in the limbic system. If the hypothalamus is thereby activated, this could explain many of the fundamental symptoms of MCS, because this gland influences the immune system, the central nervous system and the endocrine system (glands, hormones, and so forth). The limbic system is known for reacting to internal and external chemical stimulants.

Additional link: www.ei-resource. org/mcs.asp

SOURCES

B.A. Sorg et al., "Exposure to Repeated Low-Level Formaldehyde in Rats Increases Basal Corticosterone Levels and Enhances the Corticosterone Response to Subsequent Formaldehyde." *Brain Research* April 20, 2001; 898(2):31420. www.nc bi.nlm.nih.gov/pubmed/11306018?dopt=Ab stractPlus.

D.K. Sari et al., "Effect of prolonged exposure to low concentrations of formaldehyde on the corticotropin-releasing hormone neurons in the hypothalamus and adrenocorticotropic hormone cells in the pituitary gland in female mice." *Brain Research* July 2, 2004; 1013(1): 10716. www.nc bi.nlm.nih.gov/pubmed/15196973?dopt=Abst ractPlus.

NASAL PATHOLOGY AND STUDIES OF THE UPPER AIRWAYS

Several scientists concentrated on abnormalities in patients' mucous membrane and nerves in the nose and airways. Through these nerves, irritants (scents and fumes) are relayed to the brain. Researchers report increased irritation, inflammation and damage to the mucous membrane, which serves as a barrier between chemicals and the nerves. The destruction of the barrier can cause irritation or inflammation of the nerves, which causes irritants to be directed to another location through the central nervous system. This neurogenic infection can explain why, for example, inhalation of an irritant can cause ailments in places other than the airways.

W. J. Meggs, M.D., published in *Environmental Health Perspectives* an article titled "Hypothesis for the Induction and Propagation of Chemical Sensitivity Based on Biopsy Studies." It can be read online at www.ehponline.org/members/1997/Suppl-2/meggs-full.html.

More information about Professor William J. Meggs can be found on the website of the Brody School of Medicine, East Carolina University. This professor has conducted research on, among other things, neurogenic switching and its role in MCS: www.ecu.edu/ecuphysicians/DoctorInfo.cfm?ID=635.

NEUROLOGY AND BIOCHEMISTRY

Dr. Martin Pall of Washington State University uncovered the neurological biochemical processes that underlie MCS, and demonstrated a link to processes that are also relevant to chronic fatigue syndrome. He described the increased permeability of the blood-brain barrier as a result of exposure to certain substances and as a result of increased peroxynitrite level. The more this barrier disintegrates, the more chemical substances are able to directly enter the brain and the more sensitive a person becomes. Increased levels of nitric oxide in the body in turn influence the enzymes responsible for breaking down chemical substances (P450 enzyme). He published an article about his model, title "Elevated Nitric Oxide/Peroxynitrite Theory of Multiple Chemical Sensitivity: Central Role of N-Methyl-d-Aspartate Receptors in the Sensitivity Mechanism," in *Environmental Health Perspectives*. It can be read online at www.ehponline.org/members/2003/5935/5935.html.

Another source can be found at the web page of Professor Martin Pall of the School of Molecular Biosciences at Washington State University: http://molecular.biosciences.wsu.edu/Faculty/old%20files/pall/pall_main.htm.

Pall's article "Multiple Chemical Sensitivity: The End of Controversy" is available at http://www.ei-resource.org/articles/multiple-chemical-sensitivity-articles/multiple-chemical-sensitivity-%11-the-end-of-controversy. His own website: http://thetenthparadigm.org.

TILT

Professors Ashford and Miller emphasize that the cause of MCS is repeated exposure to toxic chemical substances. They prefer the term "TILT," meaning "toxicant-induced loss of tolerance," rather than MCS, and they consider TILT a condition that proceeds in two phases.

In the first phase there is exposure (repeated low doses or a single high dose) to toxic substances such as solvents or pesticides. As a result some people develop a loss of their natural tolerance. In the second phase, which in some cases manifests at a much later stage, exposures to very small doses of the same substance and different substances can result in responses at the level of multiple organ systems.

SOURCE

Prof. Claudia S. Miller, "Toxicant-induced Loss of Tolerance — An Emerging Theory of Disease?," University of Texas, *Environmental Health Perspectives*, 1997, March, 105 Suppl. 2 www.herc.org/news/ehp/miller.html

DECREASED BLOOD CIRCULATION IN THE BRAIN

SPECT scans have demonstrated that a decrease in blood circulation in the brain of some MCS patients occurs when these patients are exposed to substances like perfume. See an example at www.ourlittleplace.com/spect.html.

SOURCE

G. H. Ross, et al., "Neurotoxicity in Single Photon Emission Computed Tomography Brain Scans of Patients Reporting Chemical Sensitivities." Toxicology and Industrial Health April–June 1999; 15(3–4):415–420. www.ncbi.nlm.nih.gov/pubmed/10416294?dopt=AbstractPlus.

More theories do exist regarding the possible physical causes of MCS. The most well-known and scientifically founded theories have been mentioned. This is not intended to imply that other explanations do not hold truth; new discoveries in this field are likely. This chapter is intended to assist those interested in the scientific aspects of MCS. Perhaps it will encourage students and/or scientists to conduct further research, which will increase the chance of creating a comprehensive model. A thorough and recognized model will in turn finally allow diagnoses to be issued worldwide, clearing the way for aid and treatment for MCS patients.

28. Isn't MCS merely psychosomatic?

Besides research into the physical causes and mechanisms of MCS, research has also been conducted into the mental aspects of MCS. Almost everyone (including those who argue that MCS is a physiological syndrome) agrees that people with MCS may also suffer from mental, cognitive and emotional ailments such as depression, confusion, etc.

There are two different approaches to this conclusion:

• Some scientists argue this indicates MCS is actually a mental illness. They argue that MCS can be explained as an anxious reaction to chemicals and is a conditioned reflex, a neurosis, or a kind of mass hysteria.

• Other scientists propose that the psychological symptoms experienced by some MCS patients are not the cause but the consequence of MCS.[1] Indeed, not every patient manifests such symptoms, just as not every MCS patient has intestinal problems. There also is research which reveals that such mental symptoms only arise in circumstances of chemical exposure.[2] Similarly, those suffering from Alzheimer's disease develop an array of mental symptoms even though Alzheimer's is known to be a physical disorder.

Scientific research is available in support of both interpretations.[3] At first glance the findings thus appear contradictory, although some comments must be added to qualify this representation:

• According to a review of studies on MCS between 1952 and 1999, a majority of the studies point to physiological factors.[4]

• Scientists at Johns Hopkins University examined studies on MCS which describe the syndrome as psychogenic. They concluded that these studies often contain methodological errors, thus rendering the results "questionable" at best.[5]

• Some authors suggest that the chemical and pharmaceutical industry play a part in the continuing tendency to dismiss MCS as a psychological condition, in spite of the ever-increasing evidence that MCS has a physiological basis. Dr. Ann McCampbell, for example, wrote a damning report ("Multiple Chemical Sensitivities under Siege") chronicling the intense pressure exercised by some members of the chemical industry in order to frame MCS as a psychiatric condition, and the techniques that part of the chemical industry levied in order to influence the representation of MCS among doctors, scientists and public opinion.[6]

• Many emerging conditions (also see *entry 34*) and disorders for which existing tests do not immediately provide results and for which the causal mechanism is unknown are initially dismissed as psychological. Such was the case with multiple sclerosis and stomach ulcers, for example. Only when scientific insight into physiological causes of the condition advances and research into the physiological causes of the condition become available is this line of reasoning revised in order to conclude that a disease or condition may really be physiological. Research into MCS is currently undergoing this evolution. At the moment it can be said that while much remains unknown, the physiological mechanisms of MCS can indeed be explained in general terms. This leads Professor Martin Pall of Washington State University to say that the most important source of the controversy surrounding MCS — the initial lack of physiological explanatory models for MCS — has been laid to rest.[7]

SOURCES

1. S.M. Caress, A.C. Steinemann, "A review of a Two-Phase Population Study of Multiple Chemical Sensitivities," *Environmental Health Perspectives* September 2003; 111(12):1490–1497. www.ncbi.nlm.nih.gov/pubmed/12948889?dopt=Abstract.

2. M. Saito et al., "Symptom Profile of Multi-

ple Chemical Sensitivity in Actual Life," *Psychosomatic Medicine* March–April 2005; 67(2): 318–325. www.ncbi.nlm.nih.gov/pubmed/15784800?dopt=Abstract.

3. This link will return numerous articles from scientific journals about multiple chemical sensitivity: www.ncbi.nlm.nih.gov/sites/entrez?db=pubmed&cmd=Link&itool=abstractplus&LinkName=pubmed_pubmed&from_uid=17046989.

4. MCS Referral & Resources, "MCS Bibliography of All Peer-Reviewed Scientific Papers, Official Reports, Books and Book Chapters on MCS," www.mcsrr.org/resources/bibliography.

5. A.L. Davidoff, L. Fogarty, "Psychogenic Origins of Multiple Chemical Sensitivities Syndrome: A Critical Review of the Research Literature." *Archives of Environmental Health* September–October 1994; 49(5):316–325. www.ncbi.nlm.nih.gov/sites/entrez?cmd=Retrieve&db=PubMed&list_uids=7944561&dopt=Citation.

6. Ann Campbell, "Multiple Chemical Sensitivities under Siege," Townsend Letter for Doctors and Patients, Issue 210, January 2001. www.mindfully.org/Health/MCS-Under-Siege.htm.

7. Martin Pall, "Multiple Chemical Sensitivity: The End of Controversy." www.ei-resource.org/articles/multiple-chemical-sensitivity-articles/multiple-chemical-sensitivity-%11-the-end-of-controversy.

32. Does the media pay attention to MCS?

Articles about MCS appear with great regularity worldwide in newspapers or on television. See www.the-abc-of-mcs.com under "Articles MCS" and "Movies etc."

33. Can MCS be fatal?

There is no official register of MCS fatalities, but within MCS circles cases of death are reported (especially in the United States and Canada). These are often MCS patients who die from suicide, fatal reactions (such as anaphylactic shock or an allergic reaction) or due to complications from being unable to undergo traditional methods of treatment, such as chemotherapy. Severe MCS patients can sustain fatal organ damage. "Officially" these patients die from heart, kidney or liver failure. In these cases the cause is rarely described as MCS.

In *Part III: The Voices of Others* a section is devoted to the memory of deceased MCS patients.

34. Isn't MCS just "all in the head"?

MCS is often easily dismissed as having a psychological foundation, especially because specialists are not sure of the exact physical cause due to the complexity of the disease and the multitude of symptoms. Whenever an explanation is not immediately available for a newfound condition, the disease is often viewed as "hysteria" simply because knowledge is lacking. Other diseases as well, such as MS (multiple sclerosis), went through a process of recognition.

A good example is the story of Dr. Semmelweis. In his day and age (around 1850) he was ridiculed because he believed that after conducting autopsies, doctors should always wash their hands before assisting during deliveries. This would reduce deaths from puerperal fever, he argued, yet no one listened to him. Despite many attempts, his thesis was not accepted during his lifetime. Today all doctors agree that good hygiene is crucial.

Thus our insights and knowledge change over time. That the scientific community simply doesn't know everything is not all that strange. The human body is such a complicated and ingenious system that it's a bit premature to think we understand the system entirely. Our DNA was only recently mapped, and genetic science (and manipulation) is still in its infancy. It's completely conceivable that new diseases will arise that we do not yet see and which we do not know how to treat.

Widespread (medical) recognition of MCS will presumably not come very quickly, given that it's a very complex disease and there are probably many economic and financial interests at stake — not to mention the possible consequences for the chemical industry and our daily sense of safety, when it is officially concluded that people can get sick even from very low doses of chemical substances.

Unfortunately, perhaps the number of MCS cases must first drastically increase before serious attention will be given to MCS. Today's "canaries" must be strong in order to endure all the problems they face, because they usually do not receive much help. This is often caused by a lack of knowledge and the unthinking acceptance of public opinion.

35. Isn't MCS just a cry for attention?

There is perfect answer for this question: "If you have MCS, you're actually guaranteed little to no attention!" MCS is in fact a condition that receives very little attention.

Many MCS patients can almost never, or only with extensive precautionary measures, entertain visitors in their home. Often they are virtually unable to go anywhere and they lose their friends, family, work and thereby their whole social life. Their income from work often falls away, which worsens the financial situation. When considering all these aspects of the life of an MCS patient, MCS does not seem to me to fall under the category of "cry for attention," but under the category "seriously limiting and isolating disease, whereby the patient generally faces tribulations completely alone and must stand firm just to keep head above water." If your goal is to draw attention, I imagine you could think of something better!

PART II
The Personal Situation

Many severe MCS patients share the same range of problems, such as learning to live with loneliness, the loss of friends and family, coming to terms with wearing a protective mask in public, and so on. In this section I hope to promote the feeling in MCS patients that they are not alone, and thus provide some much-needed solace and encouragement to help them keep going and make the best of what they have.

Relatives of the MCS patient will also be able to see from this personal story that there are other people with the same range of problems who are also looking for the best way to live with this devastating and very isolating disease. By sharing the details of my own MCS story in this way I offer the opportunity of support and greater understanding to both sufferers and their families.

5

About MCS Itself

36. How did you get MCS?

Presumably a mild form of MCS has been present since my birth. A DNA test has revealed a number of inborn genetic disorders in my detoxification system. This defect may have been caused by the fact that my grandfather was a house painter and worked with solvents. I was still very young when he passed away, but now we wonder whether at the time he might have suffered from chronic toxic encephalopathy (CTE or psycho-organic syndrome), because he too had strange ailments. My father was a heavy smoker and in those days it was normal to expose small children to cigarette smoke. (Indeed, he regularly changed my diapers with a burning cigarette between his lips, because he wasn't able to appreciate my natural scents!) My body had growth problems and became deformed, and I was skinny as can be. Pediatricians had no idea what was wrong with me and my parents tried all sorts of remedies, but nothing helped. If only we had known then that more than anything else, my father's cigarette smoke likely caused me so many problems, my life would perhaps have taken a different course. My growing body was apparently unable to process the multitude of chemicals in cigarette smoke (which contains more than four thousand different chemicals!) and for this reason manifested all kinds of strange and inexplicable symptoms. A few years later, when I was about ten years old, I also regularly fell ill from exposure to chemical substances. We had come to live near a large industrial area and my mother realized quite soon that when the winds blew from the "wrong" direction I became sick, lethargic and listless. After this time my father started another job in a different part of the Netherlands, we fortunately moved to a healthy and forested area and my health improved quite a bit (although regrettably it was just for a short time of my life). In my teens I even smoked for a few years and dived headlong into nightlife. This made me very sick and lethargic and gave me other health problems, but I still did not connect them to a mild form of MCS. In 1989, when I was 28, I met my partner and moved into his old farm. This farm was a fixer-upper in a humid location, which created mold. That even mold can cause MCS and probably caused my sinus infections as well was at that time unimaginable!

My problems only started to get worse after the first sinus infection. From that moment on my health never really improved. I also began to react sensitively to cigarette smoke, exhaust fumes and smog. My inflammations became chronic, giving me more and more problems, and limited my freedom. I really couldn't go to restaurants or parties where people were smoking without paying a stiff price over the following days. The result was usually an inflamed infection and a few days of hanging around like a zombie on the couch or in bed. The zombie feeling seemed like a gigantic hangover (without having had a sip of alcohol) that just wouldn't go away.

My workplace, a truck distribution center right next to an asphalt plant, was also very unhealthy. Often the truck diesel fumes would seep into my office or the asphalt substances from the plant would blow through the open windows of the department. My colleagues had agreed not to smoke in the office, as this gave me many physical problems. One day I unexpectedly appeared at work a bit early and the room was filled with smoke! This largely answered the question of why I still came home from work with serious physical ailments and why the chronic infections didn't go away. How enormously cheated I felt! The next day, very disappointed, I quit my job. It was my first introduction to people who had no sympathy at all for my health problems and sometimes boldly lied to my face. This was just the beginning of a road paved with lack of understanding, aggression and lies when it came to simply being considerate of my health situation.

Because my sinus problems persisted, I underwent four operations to my nose within a single year, under full or local anesthesia. These anesthetics also temporarily poisoned my body and only made my reactions to all kinds of substances a lot worse. I began to react to my own perfume — and I was *very* fond of perfume.

Two weeks after my last nose operation we went on vacation in a rented RV. The RV's chemical toilet malfunctioned,

which constantly caused chemical fumes to be present in the poorly ventilated camper, making me continuously sicker. My respiratory passages had a tough time and I'd never felt so short of breath. A bad sore throat and a sudden lethargy just wouldn't pass. Only a few days later we did realize the link between the chemicals from the toilet and my health problems, but by then it was already too late.

In the following months, I began reacting severely and frequently to all kinds of synthetic substances and I constantly had serious respiratory problems, infections, signs of exhaustion; I was always short of breath. I consulted a lung specialist who could do nothing for me but prescribe inhalers and remark that I reminded him of the New York firefighters who responded to the 9/11 attacks (*see next entry*). I was still able to tolerate natural substances really well, but all chemical substances, however scant, had to be banned from my life because they continued to cause problems in my whole body. The slightest whiff of such substances made me nauseous, dizzy and shaky, and turned me into a complete zombie. My body was so poisoned (the "bucket" had overflowed), that it even began to shake and tremble. One night I awoke because I thought there was an earthquake. It took a few seconds until I realized that it was not my bed that was shaking, but me.

The time had come for drastic measures, because this was no way to live. At this time the DNA disorder in my detoxification system became known. Quarantine was the best solution for me, to give my body time to detoxify and heal. And thus the situation has stood since April 2004.

37. How did you discover your condition is called MCS?

My lung specialist set me on the right track by comparing me to the New York firefighters and rescue workers who became sick after the 9/11 attacks, showing the same kinds of symptoms. He was aware of my sensitivity to chemical substances in perfume, laundry detergents and other common products. However, he was unable to help me, because the standard diagnostic tests did not reveal anything remarkable, but I am very grateful to him for making the comparison. The lung specialist did prescribe inhalation medicine to me which first helped a great deal. Regrettably, after a while I could not tolerate these substances anymore and I had to stop using them. Instead of making me feel better the medication knocked me out on the couch.

38. Which symptoms bother you most?

The symptoms that I encounter most often are: brain fog, blackouts, infections (especially sinus infections), serious shortness of breath, problems with short-term memory, impaired concentration, irregular heartbeat, symptoms of poisoning, restless legs and a "zombie" feeling. My symptoms often resemble those of a terrible hangover and when the exposure is heavy: nausea, dizziness and trembling also come up. Although many symptoms have changed over the years and are still changing, these symptoms recur.

39. What do you do about it?

I consistently and diligently avoid all substances that will make me sick. In my case this means isolation in an MCS-safe house, eating organically and drinking purified water, purifying the air using various (portable) air purifiers, among other things. I also do not invite people who could bring harmful substances into my home and I do not go anywhere unprotected. In order to prevent infections in my sinuses and nasal cavity, I regularly squirt my own concoction into my nose and then hang my head upside down so the fluid also enters my sinuses (see *entry 286*). Usually this is able to prevent or ameliorate an infection, unless the infection is also in my lungs, in which case, of course, this won't suffice.

My condition improved greatly due to the isolation and my drastic and consistent approach, but my MCS is certainly not cured. As long as I stay away from chemical substances I'll do just fine but as soon as I am exposed to them again, I immediately become ill.

40. What do you do during acute reactions to chemicals?

First of all, the substance to which I'm reacting is removed or I remove myself from the source. In cases of acute reactions, tri-salts (see *entry 302*) or oxygen (see *entry 252*) — if I'm very short of breath — have proven helpful. Reiki treatments, deep and long meditations (see *entry 238* and *272*) or an hour-long nap also can help. This neutralizes my body's reactions. The effects are very noticeable.

41. How long does it take for the symptoms to disappear?

When the substances causing the problems have been removed, symptoms sometimes disappear right away. On other occasions it can take a bit longer and it's just a matter of patiently waiting until my liver has processed the substances; this can sometimes be a matter of days. The duration of the symptoms is strongly dependent on the degree and length of exposure. If in the meantime I've developed an infection it can even take several weeks until I'm back in shape again. In these cases I usually take a natural remedy to strengthen my immune system and overcome the infection sooner, without having to take standard medicine.

42. Did your search for a cure go well?

As stated above in *entry 36*, my problems began in the early 1990s with a severe sinus infection. The hyper-reactivity that followed has remained. Despite repeated visits to the general practitioner and the ear, nose and throat specialist due to my nose and sinus problems, little really changed: I was prescribed some inhalers, pills and antibiotics. For years I had a slightly high body temperature (99.3–100.4 degrees Fahrenheit)

because of the chronic (usually light) infections in my nose and sinuses. In hindsight the doctor was able to see this easily due to lots of scar tissue that has formed there. Only in 2002 was my problem finally recognized. I underwent a number of operations to my nose because my turbinate bone completely blocked my sinuses, causing the infections. A few years after my first sinus infection I also had the misfortune of contracting a parasitic infection while in the tropics, as a result of which I developed — three months later — severe joint and muscle pains and chronic fatigue. The general practitioner did stool analyses which provided no usable results. Because of the joint pains I consulted a rheumatologist, who officially could not ascertain fibromyalgia, because according to the research protocols two pressure points were lacking. The specialist for internal diseases couldn't help me with my intestinal and other problems.

Medically speaking I'd been turned inside out, but though I was still so ill and above all very tired, I did not want to quit my search before I knew what was wrong with me. I then continued to follow several alternative therapies, convinced of the fact that something was wrong. I thought, "If conventional medical practitioners can give no answers or solutions, perhaps alternative practitioners can give a solution." Consequently I was treated by all kinds of therapists; the most important were a bioresonance therapist, an alternative therapist and an orthomolecular nutrition specialist.

The bioresonance therapist established the presence of the parasite in my body and subsequently treated me for months (and very effectively). The alternative therapist diagnosed CFS (chronic fatigue syndrome) and prescribed for me a strict diet to combat a yeast infection in my intestines with an adjusted feeding pattern. This also turned out to be very effective. The orthomolecular therapist provided me with the necessary food and nutrition supplements. And so I was supported by a whole team of therapists working in alternative ways. The greatest thing was: it was effective! In addition, I was fully committed and was prepared to make significant sacrifices.

Due to this approach I improved and my chronic fatigue and joint and muscle pains disappeared entirely (as long as I kept following my sugar-free diet). But my nasal problems and my sensitivity stayed, no matter which therapy or theory was applied.

The first seminar I followed in support of my search for a cure was a Reiki course. This had such a deep impact on me that I practiced Reiki daily and a few years later I even gave seminars. To help myself further I learned various other alternative treatment methods as well. (You can read about these on my Reiki website, www.het-abc-van-reiki.nl/en.) Everything contributed to the fact that I kept feeling better and happier. I had discovered the power of positive thinking and with mental training I was able to free myself from a few old convictions that hampered my spiritual growth. These kinds of trainings have made me very self-aware and at the same time very strong (also see *entries 89, 90,* and *339*). Feeling content and happy has turned out to be mainly a matter of choosing which thoughts you allow to enter your mind. This has been a very important lesson in my life, from which I still benefit today.

Yet Reiki or the other alternative methods did not cure me. They healed a lot of things in me, but not my genetic disposition or the MCS I developed. Working with Reiki and meditation did give me the power and energy that I needed at the time in order to achieve many of my personal ambitions, such as giving international Reiki seminars, writing my book on Reiki, and becoming completely happy. My personal goal of finding a 100 percent cure did not succeed, but many beautiful and unexpected things came in its place. (See Chapter 9: Happy in Isolation?) Through my unrelenting quest for healing I cultivated — without at first realizing it myself— an enormous inner strength, which slowly changed the search for a cure into a daily focus on how to live with this situation. My efforts to collect knowledge about MCS increasingly came to an end and eventually were followed by a complete acceptance of and inner peace with my current situation. I became an even happier person. Despite or thanks to the circumstance I do not consider myself a victim. Yet I am happy that my search for a cure and the enduring restlessness in myself has come to an end and that now I can enjoy my life in isolation and do something worthwhile with all the information I have discovered about MCS!

43. What is your doctor's attitude towards you?

Fortunately I myself did not have too many negative experiences with doctors, perhaps because I realized rather quickly that no recognition was to be found there. A substitute for my general practitioner had made that clear by dismissing out of hand the information about the chemicals which had been used in the toilet (it was returned to me before he'd even glanced at it once), even though my symptoms coincided with the symptoms named in the document from the manufacturer. Ever since this experience I really didn't put energy into convincing or informing doctors. I prefer to leave that to the scientists. During a visit to the doctor I stick to the ailment for which I came (other than my MCS symptoms). Although it's not always easy to be taken seriously or to get attention for physical complaints other than MCS when entering the perfumed doctor's practice while carrying, for example, a mobile air purifier! By now I've switched general practitioners to one who shows more respect and understanding for my situation. In the future I plan to inform others by giving them this book, perhaps my doctor as well.

This may help other patients in the doctor's practice as well as helping myself. Above all, I just ask for respect, not recognition. This seems to work, because my new general practitioner and his assistant are willing to set aside their perfume and open the windows when I come into the practice.

44. Don't doctors generally dismiss MCS as hypochondria?

Definitely. MCS is sometimes mocked as a "fashion disease," although MCS would have been "fashionable" for quite a long time, since the early 1950s. I myself had such an experience when I placed an article about MCS on Wikipedia (Dutch version), which was immediately edited by a doctor. He added a study about food allergies, which has nothing to do with MCS. Further editing and modifications by this doctor revealed how he viewed MCS patients. After some discussion, which also involved other MCS patients, a compromise was reached. Yet the commentary from this doctor still has nothing to do with MCS. The most important thing was that MCS is listed on Wikipedia and that people can find their way to more information.

45. Do you ever go to the doctor or to a hospital?

I try to avoid doing so as much as possible, following a rule of thumb: "If something is unbearable or too painful, I'll have to go, but otherwise I'd rather not." I try to spare myself visits to the doctor or stays in the hospital as much as possible, because an extended stay in the hospital would certainly result in a serious setback to the physical improvement I have built up so far. And of course I would never enter a hospital without my air purifier.

Also see *entry 216* about the hospital protocol for MCS patients.

6

About Relationships

46. How do you and your partner deal with your disease?

Fortunately my partner is very sympathetic and understanding, although it did require the necessary investment, love, respect and perseverance from both sides (see *entry 47*). Few severe MCS patients receive understanding and sympathy, and many marriages fail because of MCS. In general MCS patients lose a lot of things in life — often their partner is one of them. The fact that my partner supports me 100 percent is a great blessing to my path! MCS rules our life, as you have to keep it in mind 24/7. My partner recognizes that as long as we uphold the protocols, things go quite well with me. The isolation, the drastic measures and the effort to keep our lives and house as chemical-free as possible, keep rewarding us both each day. When I feel good it also brings my partner great joy.

We enjoy life greatly and direct ourselves toward the things that still can be done. I also encourage my partner to keep doing things without me, such as trips, parties and other social happenings which I can no longer attend. Two people in isolation is one too many. Every now and then he takes a journey and then of course I miss him terribly. Although he never leaves for longer than two weeks, things are still very quiet and deserted and I don't see a soul. But the idea that he should therefore curtail his life and not live it to the fullest I find selfish and not an act of unconditional love.

47. How did you receive his sympathy and understanding?

A couple of things helped us greatly to understand and learn to live with MCS:

READING BOOKS AND
ARTICLES ABOUT MCS

I read a few books about MCS and had my partner read certain sections.

WATCHING MOVIES THAT
SPECIFICALLY CONCERN MCS

These movies really helped my partner, and the recognition offered by the different films and documentaries was for me a true comfort! See *Part V: Films, Books and Other Resources* for more movies about MCS and a few reviews I have written.

Final Insult, www.roninfilms.com.au/video/1871977/0/1832141.html

MCS: How Chemical Exposures May Be Affecting Your Health www.alisonjohnsonmcs.com

See *Part V: Films, Books and Other Resources* and the website accompanying this book.

DNA TESTING

Testing for the cytochrome P450 liver enzyme really created a lot of understanding. The DNA test results were explained in a very clear way by an environmental health specialist, and it made us realize that my situation was inborn and irreversible, and that we had to learn to live with it. My various ailments — which over the years had been given all sorts of names — all really fell into place after the DNA test results. It was important for me to consistently avoid chemical substances and to try to detoxify as much as possible in order to achieve improvement and prevent eventual organ damage.

DAILY EVIDENCE

My partner himself often noticed clear evidence. I'd suddenly get sick, for example, without an identifiable reason, and he'd realize that he'd just done something or experienced something which for me was unsafe. The fact that I knew nothing of it gave him confirmation that it was serious and that you have to treat MCS exceedingly carefully and keep following the agreed-upon protocols. He likes to say that while he can fool me, he can't fool my body. Because I went into isolation and we made our house completely safe (which took months to accomplish), it became easier for us to discover what exactly made me sick. These kinds of discoveries are much more difficult when you're always ill and still living in a house that elicits all kinds of reactions.

THE PAST

My partner and I knew one another for fifteen years before MCS definitively struck (after our experience with the chemical toilet in the rental RV). He realized that it did not fit my character to "choose" to have such a disease and to live in complete isolation. We were very happy and enjoyed life to the fullest. We loved going on trips and had a busy social life that gave us great pleasure. I was always up for an excursion, a party or, most of all, a dinner, and had friends aplenty to do fun things with! My great antipathy for my bad days, on which I couldn't nearly be as industrious as I would like, and my irrepressible desire to find knowledge and betterment, also made him realize that I in no way wanted this for myself. My persistence was ultimately rewarded. This did, however, mean that my life had to be turned inside out and serious sacrifices had to be made, but I would have given anything to feel well again. Anything. This confirmed everything for my partner!

LOVE

Adversity (such as health problems in both of us, a lack of contact with friends and family due to MCS) has made our relationship more special and steady. We are two pillars of strength in a none-too-sympathetic world. It's wonderful to know somebody in your life who supports you 100 percent, especially when many others fail to do the same. You yourself are also, of course, an important factor in a loving and respectful relationship. Every good relationship demands a good heart and an extensive give-and-take from both sides, even without MCS. Wanting to see each other happy and unconditionally wishing the best for one another is an important aspect of our relationship.

48. Doesn't your partner find it difficult to always go places without you?

Yes, there are certainly moments when it's very difficult for him. After all, we have chosen to share life together and that's something quite different from doing everything alone. In that regard his life has also changed drastically. In some ways he's become single. He too had to deal with a serious loss.

49. Do you experience mood swings due to MCS?

When I've had too many stimulants or exposures, it's definitely noticeable in my moods. Not only do I experience physical discomforts, but I often get irritable and that has a negative impact on my mood. Within our relationship we take that into account in order to avoid arguments, and at such times I avoid contact with others. If I don't do so it could incite stress hormones which hamper my recovery. Under the influence of chemical substances I can also be much more emotional, and I have a lot more sadness over the losses I've suffered than I do when I feel well. Without the influence of these substances I don't have such mood swings and my nature is almost always bright and optimistic.

50. Do you have children?

No, we don't have children. It would have been rather difficult to live in isolation and also be raising children who often leave the house or want to bring friends home. With just one person who goes outdoors it's already difficult enough to keep the house 100 percent safe for me. Chemical substances are of course often unintentionally brought inside. (Also see *entry 226* for information about the necessary adjustments a partner must make if he or she has been elsewhere.)

51. How did you tell your friends and acquaintances?

My social contacts largely dwindled with my withdrawal from social life, because for years cigarette smoke had already caused problems. Because of this it became increasingly difficult to go to restaurants and parties. In order to inform everyone as well and as clearly as possible, we sent a letter in which the situation at hand and the results of the DNA testing were explained. Especially for acquaintances, neighbors and others who were a bit more at a distance, this letter was very useful. In one fell swoop everyone knew why, from now on, only my partner would attend social events while I increasingly stayed behind.

52. How does your neighborhood generally react to your situation?

People who are open to explanations tend to react very well. From many people I received loving responses and they also let me know that they would be willing to do everything necessary to still be able to see me. It also makes a difference that my partner often explains the situation on my behalf (because I myself can't easily meet people anymore) using the DNA results and my website. In some cases it's even preferable for someone else to explain things for you. From an independent perspective it's often easier and simpler to convey the message. From our neighbors we get a surprising amount of understanding, for example from neighbors who call us when manure is to be sprayed on the fields (we live in a rural area) or when someone is planning to start a brush fire. This pleases us because we're then able to close the windows and doors in time and turn on our special air purifiers.

Of course, I also received less pleasant responses, such as disregard, aggression or suggestions of referrals to a psychiatrist. Naturally, I would love it if a psychiatrist could solve my problem. A pill, some therapy, and voilà, I'd get my old life back! That sounds truly fantastic — perhaps I'll swing by the travel agency on my way home! If only this was possible.

When loved ones and friends consider you mentally ill, without even caring to look into your situation, it's above all very hurtful. It's painful because apparently they don't consider you important enough to find out more about your situation, even through a book, brochure or movie. When you're a happy person with both feet on the ground and (in the eyes of others as well) a stable personality, it's odd to discover how easily people can dismiss you as "psychotic." People tend to judge others too quickly and don't take the effort to inform themselves about the person or the thing they are judging.

53. Don't people often consider MCS just a ploy for attention?

Absolutely, and they are often the same people who don't want to learn about your situation. In general it can be said that people have a hard time putting themselves in another person's situation — especially one that does not exist in their own lives. If, for example, you don't get ill from mopping the floor, it's hard to imagine that someone else would. The conclusion very quickly will be made that it's just a ploy for attention. After all, judgment is usually passed fast!

54. How does your family deal with it?

At the moment I'm not in touch with my family. In the end I was forced to break with my entire family, meaning my parents, my three sisters and their partners. The cracks in our relationships appeared when my health ailments became worse and I had to ask them be considerate of me, for example by not smoking in my presence or by ensuring that I did not indirectly inhale smoke (by airing the living room before I came over and not smoking in the doorway when I was there). Later I also had to ask them not to wear perfume. These simple adjustments turned out not to be easy for my family, so things kept going wrong. Over the years it was even a source of quarrels. These unnecessary irritations and my family's lackadaisical attitude repeatedly disappointed me and often made me return home upset and annoyed. Why did they find it so difficult to be considerate of me? It hurt me deeply when they'd say I was whining and I was once again faced with smoke or perfumes. Later, once I'd gone into isolation, their lack of willingness to make the adjustments necessary for visiting me (such as washing their clothes), really hurt me, especially because this appeared to be no problem at all for my in-laws and a number of friends. My request that they accommodate my health situation eventually resulted in sporadic and/or unprepared visits from my family. They completely failed to understand that even just a whiff of something could leave me sick for days (sometimes weeks if it inflamed my infections) and they had no idea that these symptoms derailed me so badly that I could no longer function (and how I hated those days!). My partner tried several times to explain things thoroughly and thereby engender sympathy for my situation, but unfortunately it just made things worse. The fact that chemical substances made me sick just wouldn't sink in. They didn't want to be confronted with these kind of problems, which I suppose I can somewhat understand; after all, they just wanted the "old" Els back and wanted this kind of adversity to pass them by.

The lack of understanding eventually took on such forms that my parents advised me to definitively end my relations with my three sisters. Finally I even detached myself from my parents when it became clear to me that continuing our relation put them in a tough and complicated position with regard to my sisters. Apparently not all families can hold up against MCS, although it's strange

to have to do without my parents and sisters as a consequence of my health condition.

But with MCS you simply can't continue relations with people when they show such a lack of understanding, empathy and will to make the necessary changes. With this condition it's simply impossible to pretend it doesn't exist, no matter how much we all wish it were so!

55. How do your in-laws treat you?

It's quite a consolation and a wonderful reward how respectfully my in-laws deal with the situation. They are much more open to the idea that it's possible to develop a disease that is not yet recognized in the Netherlands. They do everything they can for us to keep seeing one another and this warms my heart!

56. Have you lost many friends?

Before I started to live in isolation, I had a very busy social life. My partner and I had many friends and acquaintances and we often had to clear our schedules to avoid always being on the move. After my complete withdrawal, little is left of those days, especially for me. I can count my friends on the fingers of one hand, though the ones that remain have proven all the more valuable! My real friends stood up while my superficial friends left, never to be heard from again. The French expression "When in need, your true friends show themselves," is 100 percent applicable to my life. This filtering I now consider a fortunate side effect of my condition. After all, why waste your precious time on superficialities when you could live as intensely as I do? The few friends who remain fully accept and respect my situation, and they have no problem whatsoever making the adjustments necessary to visit me. They can't understand why people would be so narrow-minded as to refuse doing so.

57. What bothers you most?

What annoys me most are people who immediately pass judgment without first learning about the issue or the person they are judging. I'm bothered by some uninformed remarks, such as:

- "It wouldn't be worth it to me to go into isolation!"
- "Isn't it just the flu?"
- "If only you'd start thinking that you can handle it, wouldn't that help?"
- "Can't you just accept these substances?"
- "It's just a whiff, don't make such a big deal out of it!"
- "Wouldn't anti-depressants help?"
- "My perfume is a quality/expensive brand, I'm sure it won't give you problems."
- "I biked over here, so my clothes and hair will have aired out."
- "But you have a dog and a cat!"
- "My husband has an obsessive-compulsive fear of contamination and is seeing a psychiatrist; maybe that would be good for you as well."

58. What disappointed you most?

The negative reactions of people from whom you'd expect it least was my biggest disappointment. My family's reaction especially disappointed me, and I was able to accept it only after much pain and effort (see *entry 54* above).

One thing I'm still unable to understand: Why is it so difficult for people close to me (family or other loved ones) to switch to products that are safe for me? After all, the choice among laundry, cleaning and personal care products makes a world of difference to me! If they made safe choices we could keep seeing each other. Of course I could ask them this question, but I do feel a bit burdened doing so. For one thing, I'd be putting emotional pressure on them, because they couldn't any longer decently say no. And I'd also be placing a financial burden on them, because these "safe" products are often more expensive than common synthetic products. There are but few people who themselves come up with the idea to switch; most people just keep going on as if nothing is wrong (even with such radical changes in my life). It sometimes seems as if the bond between a person and their products is stronger than between two people!

59. Do you often get unwanted advice?

Nowadays I don't, but I used to get lots of it, in all shapes and sizes. Some advice was simply based on denial (such as from members of my family, who didn't want to learn about MCS but did tell me that it was all in my head and I ought to see a psychiatrist). Other offerings of advice seemed like an "over-recognition," or at least were quite remarkable, for example after I'd informed a few fellow Reiki teachers about my situation (and that I could not go to meetings anymore). A number of them advised me to receive spiritual treatment to heal my DNA disorders. And apparently I need to be (even) better grounded, because my "light bodies" are very sensitive to pollution and therefore need extra grounding. I have to learn to step right through my fears and into my strengths. Earth healings, they say, seem to help with that.

About Social Life

60. Do you still have a social life?

No, not like "normal" people do. My social life predominantly takes place online or over the phone. I go for visits only after making preparations and taking my air purifier along with me, but that's mostly in the summer so that we can sit in the yard. Going into other people's homes without my helmet is for me no longer possible (see Chapter 8: About Protective Measures), given all the chemical substances that are present in a normal home.

61. Do people still visit you?

Rarely. If people want to visit me at home, they need to strictly abide by a list of instructions, but even then it's often not 100 percent safe for me. Sometimes it's an impossible task to wash the perfume out of clothes even after a couple of washes.

Nowadays we prefer to visit others in their gardens, in which case I take my air purifier along (see Chapter 8: About Protective Measures). We have also considered setting aside a safe set of clothing for people who would like to visit us more often. They could change at our place and then approach me safely (of course they will have to use safe shampoo, deodorant, and so forth).

62. Do you have a job?

Working outside the home is of course impossible, but still we have found a way to create goals and perspectives in my life, such as building and maintaining a website and writing books. My partner earns enough to support us both, which I am very pleased about. I am very grateful to be in this situation, because many MCS patients don't have it quite so good!

63. Do you ever get to go to a party?

No, although we once held a "chemical-free" party for select company, which was wonderful. We booked a smoke-free room at a restaurant, which accommodated me fantastically. Even the staff had completely adjusted itself. The guests actually found the changes necessary to participate in the party quite doable and not a big deal. We gave everyone a set of products and a list of instructions, and this approach turned out to be a great success. It became the best night of my life. After spending a long time in quarantine I even felt a sense of regained freedom. Unfortunately it was temporary, but I had had another beautiful experience from which to draw courage.

64. Have you ever thought of moving to a different country?

Yes, for sure. But the question is: "Where to?" We have run through all kinds of possibilities, from Scandinavia, Scotland, Ireland, to the USA, Canada and the Netherlands Antilles. We drew the conclusion that wherever there are people there will be problems, even just from the combustion gases (stoves and fires, for example) and the chemical substances in the clothes that are worn. In countries other than the Netherlands social isolation would also be an issue. The availability of organic products was also an important issue for me, because in many areas — especially rural areas — they are not widely available.

The question then becomes: "How big is the sacrifice and what do you get in return?" Here in the Netherlands we live in the country and there is no industrial area nearby. Had this not been the case, we would certainly have moved. The north of the Netherlands and the islands off the Dutch coast seemed safest, but there are other (social) aspects to consider. Especially if you have a partner who has a job and a social life, he or she would be drawn along into your isolation in the event of a move to a rural area.

As long as my situation remains stable, we'll stay where we are. It's an MCS-safe house which when necessary can be well sealed and has an excellent air purifier in every room. So we hope to manage just fine in the coming years!

About Protective Measures

65. How do you protect yourself when you have to go outdoors?

I don't leave the house much but when I do, I protect myself using my portable air purifier, hose and helmet (see photographs). Often I use only the motor with the hose, but in some situations the helmet is really necessary.

66. Are there other MCS patients using such a helmet?

So far there are not many MCS patients who wear a helmet on the streets. This has to do with the following factors:

• With regard to the severity of the MCS, not everyone is at the stage where such measures are necessary.

• You have to cross a high emotional hurdle in order to show yourself in public wearing a helmet. Nobody likes to be seen as an oddity, so you do so only if there is no other way. You have to really need it.

• The system was not specifically designed for MCS and thus needs to gas out for quite a long time. The hose especially takes a while, but with patience it can be gassed out quite well.

• Some people are very hesitant because not everyone can deal well with

this system and the long-term consequences of using it are unknown. Those people are afraid that using this system will only make them more sensitive to synthetic materials and other substances (and of course if the system is not gassed out well enough before using, that could easily happen!). Those who have been using it for years say that for them this has not been the case. The system has in fact often saved them from unsafe situations (in case of environmental calamities, for example) or enabled them to do their shopping and get the kids from school. The helmet has even allowed some people to travel to areas that were healthier to them or to begin rebuilding their social lives. It's always important to take good measures before putting the device into use, as is the case with all new machines and products. For patients with mild MCS, it's of course advisable to first get their lives in order and ensure an MCS-safe home, rather than using this system right off the bat.

67. Doesn't the helmet make you feel terribly uneasy?

Yes, absolutely. There's still a great deal of shame to overcome, especially because in my youth I was taught that it's very important what others think of you. So for me it's quite a task to free

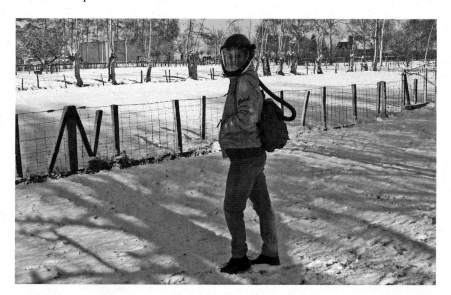

myself from this limitation. Others might have an easier time with it, but I find it awful to walk down the street like a "bubble boy." Nobody wants to be considered crazy, after all.

The song "Strong" by Robbie Williams contains a wonderful line on this subject, which inspires me to see that it's time to overcome my shame forever:

Life is too short to be afraid, step inside the sun!

My personal interpretation of this line is: *Life is too short to be afraid of what others might think of me — step outside and enjoy!*

68. How do people react to your helmet?

Everyone who is well informed about my situation thinks it's obvious that I would make use of this opportunity. These people find it impressive how well I manage to live in isolation and applaud when I once again take some steps outdoors. If doing so requires wearing the helmet, so be it. They think it's important that they can still see me, and they accept my situation unconditionally. These people react without pity; instead they encourage me to be more daring. My partner is the biggest supporter in that regard. Others apparently feel too much embarrassment over the simple fact that I need an aid such as a helmet and ban me from their lives.

69. Were you able to use the system right away (motor, helmet and hose)?

No, this system is not by definition immediately safe for use by MCS patients. I was able to use the motor and the filters after a few weeks, while the helmet needed to gas out for four months. The hose even needed to gas out for over a year. Also see *entry 274*.

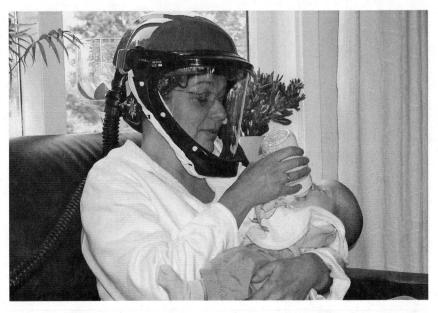

70. Can't you just use an MCS mask?

I initially made use of "normal" MCS masks. These are cotton masks with a filling of active carbon. Yet these masks are no longer effective for me; too many substances and gases still pass through and make me sick. A mild MCS patient would likely still benefit from them.

71. Would you like to travel again in the future?

If it was just the trip that would be unsafe for me, I would put on my helmet and leave right away! But it's not that simple because no matter where I go, there are chemicals. Hotels use synthetic decontaminating detergents, people use all kinds of chemical products in their homes every day (cleaning deter-gents and the like) and almost everywhere in the world there are people using synthetic care products or burning stoves or fires. In short, I'd have to walk around with my helmet 24/7, which strikes me as far from pleasant.

No, I prefer to cherish my memories, because my partner and I made wonderful journeys and have been to many spectacular places on Earth. During our RV tours we made countless bonfires on the shores of the most beautiful lakes. Sitting under palm trees, we have seen the most brilliant, romantic sunsets. We have seen other cultures, met wonderful people, made a very close foreign friend and so forth. I was able to experience it all, which keeps me going today. I'm thankful that such wonderful experiences and pictures are in my head — these at least can never be taken away from me.

9

Happy in Isolation?

72. Can MCS force you into complete isolation?

In my case that did happen. It depends, of course, on the severity of your MCS. There are many mild cases, in which people are able to tolerate several substances and for example react mainly to perfume and smoke (things that are easy for others to leave off). Not every MCS patient ends up in isolation. There are countless patients with a number of chemical sensitivities who, with a few adjustments, are able to lead a relatively normal life. I too was a mild MCS patient for many years; only later did my case worsen due to a number of unsafe and unhealthy circumstances. As a result of the lack of knowledge and a number of serious chemical exposures I was slowly forced into isolation.

73. Are you very lonely?

Sometimes I feel very alone, living much like a Tibetan monk completely secluded from the world. But I don't experience loneliness nearly as much as I do the feeling of being alone. Aloneness does not have to be something negative; on the contrary, if you are happy and comfortable with yourself, you'll find yourself in good company every day! In the past I regularly felt lonely, especially when I found myself among a group of people who failed to understand me,

didn't accommodate my health situation or even mocked me. See also *entries 84 and 86* with regard to how I entertain myself and what gives me comfort.

74. Can you be happy living in such isolation?

Definitely! It's another way of life. In the beginning you may go through a kind of grieving process due to all the losses you must process, but eventually you also learn to see the positive things about your situation. You just have to keep seeing a glass half full. It sounds like a cliché, but happiness does in large part come from the soul. I'm very grateful for the wonderful years I've had. My life is still very special and I'm still very happy, although of course I quite often long for my freedom, which I once took for granted. In *entries 88 to 90* you can read about how I draw strength and how my spiritual development and mental exercises helped me in this.

75. How did you learn to live with MCS?

By focusing on what I still have and can do in life! I can choose to fight it and consider myself a victim, or I can choose a happy and contented life. By going with the flow of life rather than struggling against it, you do learn —

even though life sometimes goes in directions you had not considered possible — to enjoy the things that come along your path.

76. Did you ever think of suicide?

Yes, there have certainly been moments that I seriously considered it. Especially when you're terribly sick (suffering symptoms of poisoning, for instance), it's not easy to maintain a joy for life. Yet the longer my isolation lasted, the better things became for me and the more these kinds of thoughts disappeared. Thanks to my spiritual awakening, which took place among other things due to years of practicing Reiki and Transcendental Meditation, I also became convinced that suicide is not the answer. It is an escape, and escaping is not part of my character. I am a fighter, so I fought for happiness and improvement until I found it. The setbacks in my life have surely made me a better person — and certainly made me a stronger one.

77. Are you afraid of dying?

No, I'm not afraid of dying at all. When my time has come I will absolutely make peace with that. To me, life and death are part of nature; it is a normal process. The hardest thing about it is letting go. MCS has forced me to let go of many aspects of my old life. I have already learned this lesson, and it helped me to overcome the fear of death.

78. Did you go through a kind of grieving process?

Of course there was a great deal of grief over the loss of my freedom, all the fun things that I could no longer do and the people who abandoned me or hurt or insulted me time and time again. How could they judge me so wrongly? Didn't they know me at all? At the same time I knew that this told me more about who they are than about me. But for every loss the rule applies: time heals all wounds!

I have nurtured my wounds, although my scars flare up at times. I hold my head up high and my shoulders straight and, despite the exodus, my life has once again become full and interesting, and I'm achieving new goals. Everyone is responsible for this themselves. It is very important to try to feel victorious, to stay there and above all not to become a victim of one's own situation. Say to yourself, "I struggle and will overcome!"

79. Have you forgiven those who abandoned you?

Yes, I harbor no grudge, anger or hate towards them. On the contrary, they are who they are, and they simply don't fit in my life any longer. They lost their spot in my circle, and that's a shame for them. Of course it's sad for me as well, but I prefer relationships based on love, openness and respect, although there may be just a few. Sometimes people accompany you on your life's path for only a small piece of it, and others for a bit longer. Evidently it's difficult for many people to completely accept and respect someone with MCS.

80. What do you miss most since you went into isolation?

I miss my daily freedom, which I once took for granted, the most. I miss unannounced visits with friends, acquaintances or family very much, or sitting on a pleasant terrace at a restaurant or coffee shop when the weather is nice, or just going shopping or going out to dinner. A day trip to a city, beach or show is also unfortunately no longer possible.

81. What are advantages and disadvantages of isolation?

One of the disadvantages is that you miss out on a considerable part of society at large. The world passes you by, especially when you also miss the six o'-clock news every now and then. And if you're not paying close attention, you very quickly become estranged from everyone. You have to make more of an effort to be part of things, albeit in a different way.

The advantages of isolation are that it can also be very liberating to no longer be under the watchful eye of society. I am no longer beholden to the social obligations that most people normally must fulfill. It seems as if life has become more pure when you are left to your own devices and almost no longer have to be concerned with others.

82. Do you ever having any outings, and how do they feel?

The things most people consider a normal outing are no longer part of my life. I do go out every now and then, such as seeing a therapist for my back — who by the way has a practice that is relatively safe for me thanks to the use of perfume-free products, and who sees me at a safe time. My partner and I also go for a ride in the car sometimes (bringing along my portable air purifier) or I pay a visit to a few friends in their yard in the summer. These are my outings and they sometimes leave me with a bittersweet feeling. On the one hand I enjoy them fully, but on the other hand I'm more prone to sadness over the fact that I can no longer do these things "normally" and that I will be viewing the world from a "fishbowl" for the rest of my life. When you've tasted "normal" life, you often are left wanting more because it tastes so nice. And then you cross the line, get too many exposures and become sick again. That can be very frustrating!

83. Doesn't the silence of isolation drive you crazy?

Noise actually drives me more crazy. Sometimes the silence can be very quiet indeed, but I only rarely have a problem with that. When that happens, I put on my favorite songs and sing along at the top of my voice. Isolation and the accompanying silence are very pure and you can become very in tune to yourself, your feelings and your experiences.

You live much more intensely in the silence than in the racket of hustle and bustle. I'd almost say (with a blink): "I wouldn't want it any other way!"

84. How do you entertain yourself?

I entertain myself primarily by writing books and poems, being active in various Internet networks, maintaining my website, doing household chores, practicing Reiki and Transcendental Meditation, listening to music, cooking and watching television in the evenings. For exercise I use my home trainer and treadmill and for relaxation I like to watch a good movie a couple of times per week. I also participate in an online movie forum where I rate and sometimes review movies. I also read a lot now that I have an MCS reading box! (See *entry 271.*) In order to get fresh air, I go outside every day and play with the dog in the fields. If there is smog or smoke in the air, I have to wear a helmet. In the summer I'm outdoors far more often than in the winter (except when there is a heat wave, which tends to result in a lot of smog). On my "zombie days" I do almost nothing and I'm bothered that I can't even do daily activities, but I just have to wait until my symptoms of poisoning and/or infections pass and my energy returns.

85. Do you manage to play some sports?

I've never been athletic. In fact I always hated sports, so I don't miss that!

Physical exercise is of course good for my body, but I do too little of it. I have a treadmill and a home trainer at home and I do use them, although I really should use them far more often!

86. What gives you comfort?

First of all, my partner consoles me by encouraging me in everything I do. I use the things that happen in my life to further develop myself and to then be useful to others, which also gives me comfort. Other things that give me consolation:

• Watching MCS movies and finding recognition in them
• Maintaining contact with other MCS patients and feeling that I'm not alone
• Listening to certain music that gives me solace, inspiration and strength, such as the music and lyrics of the following artists.

Kim Palmer, "The Dispossessed" (CD title: *Songs from a Porcelain Trailer*). Kim was a musician and an MCS patient who made amazing songs about MCS. "The Dispossessed" is one of her most beautiful pieces about MCS. (See *entries 128* and *334* for more information about her and her music.)

Robbie Williams, "Tripping" (CD title: *Intensive Care*). The words in these songs give me strength. I had similar experiences with certain people. The feeling that I will overcome is also very recognizable.

Elton John, "I'm Still Standing" (CD title: *Greatest Hits*). This music gives me strength and makes me feel good — after all, I too am still keeping my head up and am once again picking up the pieces of my life like a true survivor.

Gnarls Barkley, "Crazy" (CD title: *St. Elsewhere*). To me, the song "Crazy" is a cheerful account of the fact that people can judge you harshly, like when they call you insane. A judgment or a personal attack often says more about the person doing the judging than about the person being judged.

Listening to music is for me purely an expression of my emotions. For this reason I even like music in languages I don't understand, for then I can fill in entirely my own words and emotions to music!

87. What is most moving to you with regard to MCS?

What moves me most is when I hear yet another story of a child who has developed MCS and must deal with such huge limitations, problems and incomprehension at such a young age. A child is just starting his life, has to go to school, make a career, find a partner, start a family and so on. These normal life events are in some cases very difficult or even impossible for young MCS patients, which breaks my heart. When I learn of a new case of MCS my reaction is usually very emotional. I cry for these young "canaries" and how early they lost their freedom.

88. Do you seek strength in faith?

I am convinced that there is more in life than what we can see or experience

with our naked eye, and I draw great strength from this. Often I've felt that there is a wondrous, invisible and clearly perceptible force in my life. You must live life yourself and you are responsible for your own choices and decisions, but I absolutely do feel loving support in everything I do, and it doesn't come from my partner and me alone.

In order to experience this I don't need any church or specific religion. I prefer to keep myself far from such institutions. The past and the present demonstrate to me too many negative consequences of the various beliefs and groupings in the world, while in my opinion we're all actually saying the same things with different words.

89. What has your spiritual path done for you?

My background and experiences have given me a spiritual awakening, and I'm able to draw great strength and wisdom from my "inner source." It's also my conviction that things always happen for a reason. Many events in my life which first made me feel like a victim really had to happen. Setbacks sometimes turned out to be blessings on my path. I'm convinced that I have a kind of task here on Earth and that my situation and life have a special purpose. Such thinking gives me courage and above all the confidence to keep going, even if I may not yet know the full reason or purpose of all this.

90. What exactly did the mental exercises do for you?

During my spiritual development I found that you can influence your life, your emotions and your feeling of happiness just through your own power of thought. Because I struggled with my health for years I began researching this as well, hoping that my own power of thought could heal me. Although I did not cure my MCS, I gained a great deal from these exercises. They freed me from a number of negative convictions in my life and replaced them with positive convictions. This by itself was already a very big step towards happiness. The journey taught me that you can consciously block out certain thoughts not by fighting them but simply by focusing on other, more positive thoughts. At first it was a struggle, and every day I practiced affirmations (positive confirmations that you repeat multiple times per day to "reprogram" yourself, as it were), but now it comes automatically. I now immediately notice when I allow poisonous thoughts to enter my mind. As soon as I become aware of this, I let the negative things go and keep on going with a good and happy attitude. A useful exercise can be found in this book: *Empowerment: The Art of Creating Your Life As You Want It*, by David Gershon and Gail Straub. (Also see *entry 339*.)

91. How do you see your future?

Nowadays I live exclusively day by day and don't think too far ahead. A pleasant kind of emptiness has taken its place in my mind. Perhaps this is the "enlightenment" that the alternative thinkers speak of. But when I look to the future of our planet, I'm not too hopeful. Not for MCS patients, but also not for the rest of humanity or fauna and flora. We're making a mess of things. What a terrible inheritance to leave behind for our children — and this is an inheritance that can't even be refused, it'll be handed to them just like that! The thought that I might become much sicker is not too comforting either, and if my partner passes away, I'll be living completely alone and 100 percent secluded. So surely you will understand, dear reader, that I'd like to skip to the next question now.

92. Do you still speak to fellow MCS patients?

Yes, I regularly "speak" to other MCS patients over the Internet. Often it's a matter of help and information, but some contacts also have become more friendly and personal.

93. What is your advice to other MCS patients?

Despite everything, try to stay happy and enjoy life and, if you have a partner, each other. Being happy is easier when you feel physically well, so make sure that you drastically adjust your life to MCS. If you are feeling physically improved, it will make a world of difference for your state of mind. The road to improvement is usually long and difficult, but if you persevere and keep figuring out the causes of your physical reactions and above all are prepared to make real sacrifices to find improvement, you're on the right track. The art of happiness is to go along with the changes in your life and always try to make the best of it, like enjoying the small things still present in your life.

The fact that happiness comes mainly from the soul seems like a cliché, but I really do experience it this way.

Reiki and meditation have strongly supported and developed this awareness in me, and I advise everyone to adopt these practices, even if only because it helps neutralize your physical reactions to chemical substances!

PART III
The Voices of Others

The author is not responsible for the statements and opinions expressed in the personal stories of the various MCS patients. These stories are also not intended to point to something or someone as being guilty, but simply to show how MCS patients fell ill and how their lives are now.

10

Owners of International Organizations and Websites

94. Lourdes "Sal" Salvador, 38, USA

Founder of www.mcs-america.org, www.mcs-hawaii.org

My life was ordinary. I worked for 20 years, flying from Hawaii to California five times per year for meetings, before I slowly descended into the depths of darkness. I did not know what was wrong. I was suddenly very tired all the time and in the mornings did not wake up refreshed. My hair was dull and falling out in clumps. My skin was dry and scaly and constantly itchy and I had gut problems. My vision blurred almost constantly and I often felt dizzy. I developed night sweats so badly my bed would be soaking wet, as though someone turned a garden hose on me while I was sleeping. I suffered tachycardia (a form of cardiac arrhythmia) and nearly blacked out in the shower several times when my heart rate would suddenly change in the morning.

My friends thought I was making excuses and did not want to see them, because I looked healthy. They did not understand how fatigued I really was and they gradually drifted away. I moved from job to job, sleeping more and more, feeling like I was losing my mind, and then starting to have what doctors might call panic attacks (had I reported them). I knew they were not

panic attacks as I had no reason to be panicked nor had I any history of depression or anxiety of any sort. I've always been a very decisive type who knows myself well. My gut told me something was physically very wrong, seriously wrong.

I'd seen 30 doctors or so, none of whom examined me more than checking my heart rate or looking in my ear. Each tried to convince me I was depressed and told me to go on antidepressants, which I fortunately refused; I later found out that strong backbone of mine may have saved my life, as those drugs could have made me very ill indeed (as is evident from the experiences of other MCS patients).

I began chelation therapy without questioning what harmful side effects this might have. I was so relieved to have a reason for my ills beyond "it's all in your head" when I knew something was physically wrong with me! I chelated seven days a week year round as it was the only way to keep myself out of bed. I did not know at the time how damaging it was or how hard it was on my adrenals and liver.

I think I had MCS tendencies all along and that perhaps mercury poisoning and/or chelation therapy pushed me over the edge into full-blown MCS. At any rate, after I finished my chelation therapy I developed a heightened sense of smell which slowly led to brain fog, confusion, reactive airway disease, and bronchial spasms when I am exposed to any type of chemical, including fragrances, pesticides, and laundry products.

With the little money I had I could not afford a place with a washer and I began going to the Laundromat, where I often felt overcome by the fragrance of the laundry soaps and fabric softeners when clothes were in the dryer. I would often stand outside while I waited. Eventually I noticed tremors if I did not retreat outside soon enough, and soon I had my first seizure. The tremors hit hard and I dropped the laundry I was folding onto the floor and stumbled toward the door to get outside. It was too late. When I woke up the ambulance was there and I was told I'd had a seizure. I had several seizures over the next few months, and each happened at the Laundromat. Sadly it took me over a year to make the connection to the laundry products causing my problems. I stopped going to the Laundromat but it was too late. The damage was already done. Now simply being near people who used any type of commercial laundry product on their clothes triggered my seizures and I sank into the depths of isolation from MCS.

In order to subscribe to the monthly newsletter *MCS America News*, send an e-mail to subscriptions@mcs-america.org

95. Alison Johnson, 67, USA

Writer, editor, filmmaker and proprietor of www.alisonjohnsonmcs.com

Chair of the Chemical Sensitivity Foundation: www.chemicalsensitivityfoundation.org

My daughters and I are among the lucky people who developed MCS and have recovered sufficiently to be able to live our lives without excessive restrictions. There was no obvious exposure that made us all sick, and the reasons why each of us developed MCS years apart are not at all clear. My surveys and extensive personal contacts with people with MCS, however, have indicated it is highly likely there is a genetic predisposition toward developing MCS. Nevertheless, it appears to me that almost anyone can acquire MCS, given a sufficiently large exposure to a toxic substance.

One of my first major exposures to chemicals occurred when I was about eleven. I slept right next to our coal furnace and, thinking back, I remember that this was a period when I had constant colds and bronchitis. Years later, when I got married, I once again had some extensive exposures to chemicals. I loved New England antiques, and over the next six years I refinished at least eighteen pieces of furniture. I removed coat after coat of paint with paint stripper, which is a fairly potent solvent. It was too cold outside for the paint stripper to work. So although the labels on the cans said to use with adequate ventilation, I would open a window a few inches and do the work inside, exposing myself to the toxic fumes.

When my husband and I bought an older house, we also did all the redecorating work that we were capable of doing ourselves. For months we were breathing toxic fumes. One other exposure that I've sometimes wondered about occurred when my husband and I spent a few months in Paris. I have a clear memory of walking into the kitchen every morning and flinging open those tall French windows to let in as much fresh air as possible because I could smell gas fumes.

The next winter, back in the States, I happened to have a fairly heavy exposure to cigarette smoke because I was on a committee that met in my kitchen a couple of nights a week. One member was a heavy smoker and would smoke six or seven cigarettes in the course of the evening. That, of course, was back in the days when you didn't dare ask anyone not to smoke in your house. That March I had pneumonia, and about three weeks after I recovered from that, I began having migraine headaches for the first time in my life (I was thirty-three). After I'd had several of these migraines, I made the connection that they always started after I had been exposed to heavy cigarette smoke the previous evening. Sometimes there was a ten-hour delay between the exposure and the reaction. After a few months, I also began to see that exposure to heavy diesel fumes could trigger a migraine.

Back in 1972, when I first experienced clear symptoms of chemical sensitivity, there was virtually no information available on the subject. At last I found out about the work of Theron Randolph, M.D., whose book *Human Ecology* I found to be very helpful. It was a great relief to find someone at last who understood the unusual condition I had developed. In the early 1970s, far fewer therapies were available than the wide variety today. My only option was to avoid chemical exposures and problem foods, which still seems to be the most effective way for me to recover some degree of tolerance. I started using as many organic food ingredients as I could, I drank spring water to avoid chlorine and I decided to go on a rotary diet, which I followed for about a year. When I temporarily eliminated certain foods and drinks from my diet and avoided cigarette smoke for a year, my migraines disappeared.

My husband and I decided to make major changes in our home to reduce my exposure to chemicals. We also went through the usual MCS routine of changing over to less-toxic cleaning products, laundry detergent, and personal care products. I am grateful to my husband, who never questioned the reality of my chemical sensitivity. Like me, he was ready to look for cause and effect. When I had a reaction, the question was what I had eaten or been exposed to, not whether I had had a stressful day.

There is virtually no physical symptom I experience that I can't trace to an exposure to a chemical or food. I have recovered from MCS to a large extent, but I still have to be aware of my underlying chemical sensitivity. At this point, however, it places no great restrictions on my life.

When our daughters began, one at a time, to develop MCS a few years later, we recognized the symptoms right away. We were able to immediately ask them the right questions and discover the cause of the problem. It wasn't easy raising daughters with MCS, but we kept them healthy enough to be starters on their basketball teams, and they eventually got degrees from Harvard and Yale law schools. One reason they have been able to stay healthy is that they always look for apartments with hardwood floors, electric stoves, and hot-water radiators. Although my daughters have been leading normal lives for some time, they can maintain this status only by rigorously avoiding exposures to substances they know have caused problems in the past.

Avoidance of exposures has been the one thing that has worked to return all of us to health. We each still have some chemical sensitivities, but we can work around them well enough to live full and productive lives.

Also see: www.conceptmed.com/Johnson/mcs1/mcs1.html

Alison Johnson has produced various books and films. See *Part V: Films, Books and Other Resources.*

96. Peggy Troiano, 64, USA

Founder of MCS Beacon of Hope: www.mcsbeaconofhope.com

My husband, Domenic, and I became very ill shortly after moving into in a new residence. We did not realize at that time there were toxic chemicals leaking, out-gassing and contaminating our air. Shortly after moving into this recently remodeled property, we started noticing strange odors, sometimes light but offensive, sometimes strong, sometimes unbearable. We didn't know that we were being exposed to formaldehyde, toluene, mold, asbestos, fuel oil and other toxins. In the beginning, during an absence from the home we would notice some improvement in our symp-

toms, but upon returning home we would very soon be as ill or worse than before. This happened for a while, but then the time came when there was no improvement even upon leaving the home.

Soon, we started to also experience adverse reactions to odors and fumes from all kinds of chemical substances, such as perfume, gasoline, and the detergent aisle in the grocery store. The deodorants, soaps, shampoos, clothes and other household and cleaning products that we had used before were now causing us to become very ill. We would break out with rashes and my hands would crack open and bleed. Domenic and I would experience great difficulty breathing. It was as if an eighteen-wheeler had parked on our chests. We became so ill that we could no longer enjoy going out to eat, shop or socialize. It was a daily struggle just to survive.

Life became like walking on a minefield. That house and its toxins had turned our lives into a living hell. Life as we once knew it was gone! As time went by we had more and more symptoms, including but not limited to head, body, and joint aches and pains; skin rashes and dermatitis; never-ending flu-like symptoms; dizziness, extreme fatigue, and respiratory problems; mental confusion and short-term memory lapses; increased sensitivity to sound, light, colors and patterns; bloating and other intestinal problems; heart palpitations; lack of coordination, stroke-like symptoms, and others too numerous to list.

I spent years watching Domenic struggle with the senseless pain and suffering caused from what could have and should have been avoided. Then tragically and unnecessarily, Domenic's life was prematurely ended. On January 3, 1999, a snowy winter's day, I very unexpectedly lost my soul mate, the love of my life and the father of my children. We will always mourn the loss of his life, his presence, his laughter, his singing and his hugs. Our children and I also miss the person that I was before those toxic exposures completely devastated our lives as we lost a wonderfully loving and compassionate husband and Pop, and I also lost my health and my freedom. I've been forced into living in isolation with constant pain. I have upper and lower reactive airway dysfunction, brain toxic encephalopathy, fibromyalgia, and chronic fatigue, along with other serious health issues.

Much pain and suffering has been forced into our lives by the careless acts of others and many tears have been shed: tears for what was and will never be again; tears for all the hopes and dreams that were permanently destroyed; tears for all that was so precious to us having been senselessly taken away; tears because this tragedy could have and should have easily been prevented.

As our conditions continued to deteriorate, Domenic and I made a promise to one another that if the Good Lord did not call us home together that whoever remained would do all they could to prevent this horrible tragedy from happening to other families. The loss of our health, family, friends, independence, economic productivity, the health of our environment and natural resources will only continue to worsen if we do not do something about it ... now!

Water was always very important to Domenic and still is to me. Besides being a very talented carpenter, Domenic had a captain's license and was also a fisherman. We made our living off the New England waters. Our foundation's name, MCS Beacon of Hope, is in memory of Domenic and our love for the ocean. The lighthouse beacon signifies the way out of despair, a shining hope for those living with chemically/toxically induced illnesses and to let them know someone cares and is working to bring hope, help and solutions back into their lives.

Peggy and Domenic's story can also be found online at www.mcsbeaconof hope.com/our_journey_into_toxic_inju ry2.htm

97. Julie Genser, 40, USA

Founder: www.planetthrive.com

My life was derailed by extensive food and chemical sensitivities brought on by exposures to multiple environmental toxins. During my twenties and thirties I was exposed to a broken mercury thermometer, a toxic garbage dump fire, the harmful fumes (and emotional trauma) from the World Trade Center fires of 9/11, and mold resulting from a flood in my apartment. Finally, I tested positive for Lyme's disease, which I believe has been underlying all of my other health challenges for over thirty years. My symptoms have included a wide range of respiratory problems (shallow, labored breathing, swelling of my tongue and throat, sleep apnea, shortness of breath), migraines, digestive disease, brain fog, depression, anxiety/panic, inability to handle stress, and more.

I first became aware I had MCS in

September 2004 during a nightmare that unfolded in Washington State and Arizona. Local conditions — mold, pollen, daily controlled forest fire burnings, pesticides — brought on severe MCS, and along with it, post-traumatic stress disorder (PTSD).

Before I had MCS, I spent a full year backpacking around the world. I was passionate about photography. I was a freelance writer for a holistic company. I was crafting my life to support my dream of living a nomadic lifestyle. MCS has been a very hard condition for me to accept because of my deep nomadic yearnings. MCS restricts one's lifestyle like nothing else. Imagine feeling like you suddenly can't breathe, but all the triggers are invisible. It's like being a blind detective. We have to rely on our heightened sense of smell and the sensitive meter our body has become to figure things out.

What happens is that you create as safe an environment as you can in your home, and then you rarely leave it. I've really had to develop my inner life — my dreams, my memories, my online relationships — in order to feel satisfied with my life on a daily basis. And I do. I've never really felt as content as I do now. Part of that has been reevaluating my expectations and finding acceptance in "what is." Another part has been slowing down and nurturing myself. But the biggest shift for me was hitting rock bottom mentally and having to rebuild my view of the world — a world that I had some control over.

That's where my website Planet Thrive comes in. Most of my health research was done online, where I found anecdotal information and support from

others dealing with the same issues — a real life-saver for me after being misdiagnosed and dismissed by doctors for years. There are millions of others doing the same. Planet Thrive is for them. We create a fertile space catering to mind, body and spirit where people are more than their illness — and help them to start making the connections between our environment, government, big business and our health. We believe that illness is not an unfortunate hand we are dealt in life, but is an opportunity to learn from a great teacher. We strive to harness the collective intelligence that comes from the lessons illness brings us.

98. Susan Abod, 55, USA

Producer of the film *Funny, You Don't Look Sick*, www.susanabod.com/videos.html

In 1986 I was diagnosed with chronic fatigue immune dysfunction syndrome (CFIDS) and my whole life as I knew it changed. Before I got sick I was a word processor during the day, and after work and on weekends I was singing professionally in clubs and concerts and teaching music. But after I got sick I was spending most of my time in bed.

When my doctor first told me over the phone that I had this virus, I was elated! That may sound odd, but I was so relieved; now I actually had something confirmed, why I felt so wiped out for all these months, wondering if I was making this all up. So I wasn't crazy!

Soon I began to notice I was becoming more sensitive to smell. Every time I went to the movies or to public events, it seemed that someone who had a lot

4

In Conclusion

29. How many MCS patients are there?

MCS came into being alongside the growth of the chemical industry. In the early 1950s Dr. Theron called it environmental illness; see *entry 12*. Over time it was found that a relatively large group of people in society could not or could barely tolerate chemical substances. The number of diagnosed MCS patients in the United States is estimated at approximately 3 percent of the entire population, and 12 percent of those questioned in a survey stated they react sensitively to various everyday chemical substances. The California Department of Health Services even estimates 15 percent of the population suffers from chemical sensitivities. These are, of course, startling figures to have arisen in such a short time, over a few generations. At the link www.pubmedcentral.nih.gov/articlerender.fcgi?toolispub med&pubmedid=15117694, you can read the article "Prevalence of Multiple Chemical Sensitivities: A Population-Based Study in the Southeastern United States," published in 2004 in the *American Journal of Public Health*.

30. Where should I go if I think this book pertains to me?

In case of health complaints it's first advisable to consult your general prac- titioner or doctor. This is not a medical book, and you certainly should not undertake steps that would obstruct medical help. When all other possible physical causes of your health condition have been ruled out and, given this information, you really are convinced that you are an MCS patient or that the source of your sensitivity lies in the realm of chemical substances and scents, you should — besides finding an environmental health specialist (see *entry 15*) — thoroughly study up on the subject. The more knowledge you have, the more effective measures you will be able to employ in your life, and eventually improvements will be made. In *Part VI: Further Resources*, many organizations are listed, including several online MCS groups you can join. Also see *entry 15* concerning environmental health centers and lists of physicians.

31. Where can I find more information about MCS?

Aside from this book, a lot of information can be found on www.the-abc-of-mcs.com. A sort of "yellow pages" for MCS, this site has a multitude of links to national and international, extensive and informative websites. This website, which went online on May 10, 2005, accompanies this book and was constructed by the author. It is regularly updated.

of perfume or after-shave on would always wind up sitting right next to me. A few minutes later, I'd get a throbbing headache and a sore throat that was searing dry and burning. My legs would start to feel heavy. It was like they were being held down with weights. I wondered if I'd be able to drag myself home. Then I started to notice that every time I used my gas oven I lost my ability to concentrate. I'd find myself standing in the middle of my kitchen, trying to think of what to do or say next.

I didn't put any of this together until a friend came over and told me my gas stove made her sick. She said she was chemically sensitive. Her symptoms sounded so much like mine that I went to her doctor, a clinical ecologist. Test results showed I had abnormal levels of chemical substances in my blood. Somehow these chemicals got inside me and were now affecting my immune system. That's when I was told I had Multiple Chemical Sensitivity and now, like so many others, my lifestyle was to completely change. Thus began my long journey.

Since I couldn't consistently keep up with part-time work and also do the basics of taking care of myself, such as grocery shopping and laundry, focusing on my healing became my priority. One of the first actions I took was going to a support group. I went on welfare and food stamps and Medicaid while I endured the one-and-a-half-year process of qualifying for disability, which I received after the third appeal.

I talked to others who have MCS and followed their lead about what services are available to people with disabilities. I found out about and applied for fed-

eral housing assistance and started searching, searching, searching for a safe, accessible place to live. It took over two years to find an apartment and a landlord that would take the certificate. For over three years I lived just dealing with basic survival needs: shelter, food, medical help, clothes.

Seven years later, during a time when I was very sick, I saw a documentary that inspired me and I got a very strong desire to make a video about my experience with CFIDS and MCS. I knew nothing about the medium, but I got out of bed and wrote a synopsis in a half-hour. Three years later, with the help of a few very dedicated volunteers and technical crew, *Funny, You Don't Look Sick: An Autobiography of an Illness* was showing at a museum in front of two hundred people! The completion of *Funny, You Don't Look Sick* far exceeded my expectations and gave me a new way to express my creativity.

During the final editing of *Funny You Don't Look Sick*, I realized how much we needed another video to expose the proliferation of MCS and the frightening variety of different causes for its onset. I especially wanted to explore the vital issue of safe housing as treatment and prevention for MCS. My own battle with housing has been, and continues to be, so difficult. For example: In 1996 my landlord unwittingly put down treated cedar chips right under my first floor windows. I was forced to leave immediately. I was lucky enough to be able to stay at an MCS friend's house on her tiled kitchen floor until the chips were removed. A year later, the owner of my apartment wanted me to vacate because she was selling the building. I had to get a court order extension for twelve months in order to stay in a safe place while looking for another.

It was the beginning of an exhaustive housing search that lasted over three years and eventually brought me to Santa Fe, New Mexico. I am one of the lucky ones because through it all, I've been able to stay indoors. Others have not been so lucky and are living in an RV or outside. I wanted to find out how many others were going through this nightmare as well, and how did they get sick? Were they having as much trouble as I was finding and keeping a safe place to live? How were they coping with such an overwhelming and often isolating condition? Was one area of the country safer to live in than another? All these questions form the basis of my new film, *Homesick: Living with Multiple Chemical Sensitivity*. An eight-minute video trailer can be seen at www.homesick-video.com.

Today, I am still sick with MCS but I am slowly getting my life back since moving into my current house. I just applied to the Division of Vocational Rehabilitation in hopes of being able to start working part-time (most likely from home). I am occasionally performing again. However, just this past month I have been in a CFIDS episode and my MCS reactions increase when this occurs. It has put a halt to most activities and I've been feeling very discouraged. And so it goes.

99. Diana Buckland, about her son James, 18, Australia

Founder: MCS Global, www.mcs-global.org

I myself am not diagnosed with MCS — it is my eighteen-year-old son James. So I am the global warrior who does not have MCS but who is fighting for recognition for others.

My young son's health was damaged by chemicals (in particular pesticides, insecticides and herbicides) and he was affected both mentally and physically. As an infant James had a major exposure to pesticides and he had severe reaction to vaccinations when he was four months old. Also, we had a flea plague here and our home was sprayed. He became very ill. When he was eighteen months old our home was renovated and painted with the "normal" toxic paint products. He continued to have exposures at school. I had no idea they were fogging the trees and around the classrooms with pesticides. At school he was also exposed to toxic paint products and cleaning products, chemical deodorizers in the toilets and chemically perfumed products on the staff and children.

James was getting sicker and sicker and his behavior continued to deteriorate. He was violent, psychotic and suicidal and would go into destructive rages. He said the headaches were killing him, that he couldn't stand it and didn't want to live. He would vomit a lot, had gastric problems at times, had awful skin rashes and irritations, an itchy nose, and black rings under his watery, sensitive eyes. He was pale and thin and also suffered problems with his hearing. The medications (there were lots) made him more toxic, especially the asthma medications. I noticed his allergies and sensitivities getting worse! Due to his health problems James has been out of school since the age of ten. We live in isolation from the community and family as there are chemicals and chemically perfumed products everywhere — and no one cared or believed what we said.

When you do find out through the doctors practicing environmental medicine what is wrong with your child (or yourself) and you need to avoid all chemical exposures (including chemically perfumed products), in most cases your family and friends are unwilling to comply — so you're in a "lose-lose" situation.

When I keep James away from chemicals and chemically perfumed products and of course all food and drink containing chemicals, he has no more asthma. He is doing much better now at eighteen but is very lonely and of course, with no education, does not have much of a future to look forward to. I applied for a disability pension for James which was granted in July 2004.

If only we had access to health care and education and social facilities that were chemical-free and perfume-free, people with allergies and chemical sensitivities would have some quality of life.

100. Graham Guthrie, 54, Australia

Founder, sauna detox group

Like so many others I never thought twice about the dangers of using chemicals. I never used masks or protective clothing when using herbicides and pesticides. The sprays I used are more toxic than cigarettes, but while they warn us about cigarettes they never warn us about herbicides and pesticides. What

kick-started my MCS was making chicken nesting boxes out of herbicide drums, which a farmer had suggested and said was safe — so I washed them and cut them. After this I started to get sensitive to furniture polish and shower cleaner, perfumes, et cetera. I would get very angry and hard to live with. I started getting bronchitis every year.

One day I was welding my trailer when a smell was overpowering my welding. I stopped to realize there was a guy spraying the foundations for a new home across the road. The spray was coming straight over onto me, so I went inside. Within a fortnight two trees died that were next to where I was welding. I found out later he had to have herbicide mixed in with the pesticide to do that. Around that time I started to get very ill and had really bad diarrhea. My doctor had me on antibiotics for months to stop the diarrhea. I also went through six weeks of shakes and hot and cold sweats. It took two years to realize I had chronic fatigue syndrome (CFS). That started sixteen years ago.

Six years ago I got poisoned by a new antidepressant my doctor gave me, which set me off into Multiple Chemical Sensitivity. I got the shakes and was crying and experienced all sorts of weird side effects. I went on different tablets, but things then got even worse. Things got so bad I really thought I was going to die. I started to hurt all over, my skin got sensitive, my teeth started to really hurt and break down, my throat was raw all the time and I could not stand having any chemical at all in the house. I got polyps in my nose from using a tissue and I had all my teeth removed.

So by then I'd become a severe MCS

patient. After researching, the only thing I could find to help rid the toxins was a sauna, so I started to use the local gym's sauna. I started to pick up quite well and a lot of my symptoms totally disappeared, but I also started to get side effects as I was not replacing enough salts like magnesium, potassium, and calcium. I had to have a heart operation to stop my arrhythmia; the surgery did not work, and later I realized it was lack of tri-salts (see *entry 302*) that caused the arrhythmia. I also helped a few people that had to have the same operation — I told them what happened to me, they all tried taking extra salts and their arrhythmia was gone. I decided there must be a lot of other people like us going through the same nightmare of having to go to hospital for no reason (which is especially rough for MCS patients).

I made a sauna detox group to stop others from making the same mistakes. The group has helped lots of people. I did not know what I would have done without the great people in my group; they have helped me too. I believe using the sauna has saved me and I see light at the end of the tunnel. All of the following things have improved or totally gone since using a sauna: blood pressure, light and sun sensitivity, vertigo, circulation problems, poor energy and concentration, sore throats, sinus problems, bronchitis, anger, depression, poor vision, night sweats, insomnia, sleep problems and restless legs. I can now go to a lot more places than I could six years ago.

Graham's blog with a picture of himself and his son: http://grahamsback yardpics.blogspot.com

101. Season BubbleGirl, 26, Australia

Proprietor, www.bubblegirl.net

I had no symptoms of MCS until ten years ago when I was sprayed in my face with deodorant. My boyfriend held me down while my neighbor sprayed an entire can into my face. Many feel this was abusive, but really it was just imitating what students at school had done to other students. When my mother came in from putting out the washing, she stopped them immediately, furious at their immaturity. But we never thought punishment would go beyond that. Within a few hours I could not speak, breathe normally or remain awake, and I was shaking all over. My family took me to the hospital and an eight-hour session in the emergency room followed. Yet the doctor said this was a once-off situation and would not happen again. Unfortunately they were wrong. I had a secondary attack the next day and another four instances followed, forcing us to realize it might no longer be possible to continue a normal life.

The reactions were diagnosed as anaphylactic shock, a common allergic reaction among bee sting victims, for example. Mine is harder to control because of the popularity of perfumes, fragranced products, cleaners, toiletries and cosmetics, car fumes, fertilizers, and the thousands of items that can cause my vocal cords to swell and my body to go into shut-down mode.

Isolation is thought of as difficult, but when compared to deadly bouts of anaphylactic shock, it is the best option. My doctors and mother knew this when they removed me from school to stay home in a sterile and protected environment. All chemicals had to be exterminated from the home, including the carpet which had been treated with deodorizers and colorants. Sometimes I tried to live a normal life and ignored or belittled the possible consequences. Once I tried to have a friend visit, which ended up in their having to leave after my throat closed up, convulsions began and a full-blown anaphylactic attack had occurred. I later found that my friend had worn deodorant when asked not to. This added fuel to the debate over whether MCS is real or not: I didn't even know she'd broken a rule until my immune system began to "overload." Since then friends have not visited me because they cannot become "sterile" and chemical-free enough to enter the home. Instead, I enjoy friendships over the phone and Internet with people I truly adore. My best friend in Illinois and I enrich each other's lives more than other friendships we have.

Due to my illness we have had to make adjustments to our home. The most unusual improvement is the see-through plastic shield between the office and rest of our home. The computer is situated in this room, the cords going through the walls to the monitor, keyboard and mouse which I can use. Essentially, the computer is split up between the dangerous part (the computer's housing and the discs) and the safe parts (the monitor, keyboard, and mouse) which were carefully selected and detoxified by long hours of gassing out and vinegar washes. When I want a particular disc or DVD, my father places them into the computer's CD/DVD drive for me, to avoid my

being exposed to the print and chemicals involved in the disc's manufacture. Many things are still possible thanks to the presence of this plastic wall. Computers are a lifeline to me for shopping, friends, research, my website, and writing and craft pursuits.

Almost ten years later, I do not regret what my boyfriend (at the time) and neighbor did. The stupid ideas often bred in schools are not intended to be potentially deadly to the victim. (Other students had not reacted as seriously as I had, as scientists believe MCS is dependent on genetics as to how severe it becomes.) I now concentrate on my writing (books, novels, articles), website, craft (punch needle embroidery, knitting looms, butterfly looms, sewing, knitting, crochet) and musical instruments (flute, recorder, tin whistle, fife). Rising above our difficulties is a real journey, but one I have completed without emotional scars. Once the grieving period had passed, as sufferers must grieve for what they once had, I pulled myself together to become an inspiration and motivation to others with MCS.

Everyone is welcome to my website, www.bubblegirl.net, to learn about the disease and the hundreds of chemical-free hobbies and routines that will make their lives more rewarding and functional.

Season BubbleGirl is the author of *Absolute Individual: Life in a Bubble*, available on www.amazon.com

102. Helle Kongevang, 50, Denmark

Proprietor, www.mcshelle.dk (also in English)

Helle also features in the documentary *Chemical Kids* (see *entry 317*)

I have had MCS ever since I was born and have thus been ill for my entire life. I was born with a poorly functioning immune system, which doctors tried to strengthen with bacteria injections, to no avail. In 1984 the chemical sensitivity began worsening. My asthma returned (I was born with asthma and all kinds of allergies) and I began reacting to various things. In August 1992 it got so bad I could no longer work — and I never went back. In 1994 I had the lowest possible welfare aid and after a seven-and-a-half-year battle against the Danish social security system, writing letters and employing a lawyer, I won the case. I received the highest possible payout and was declared 100 percent disabled. Now I live on Fano, a small island off the west coast of Denmark. This brought great change in my life — this time for the better. I have never felt this good, not even in the period before I got so sick!

MCS can still suddenly make me very sick, usually when we leave the island. Because I have MCS I wear a mask (you can see a picture of me with my mask on, on my website). If I don't wear it I get severe reactions as soon as I am exposed to triggers. The reactions vary with different substances, and if it turns out to be a cocktail of substances, the most bizarre things can happen. My reactions can be: heavy respiratory problems, a choking sensation, vomiting, migraine, dizziness, a loss of memory, speech and hearing problems, crying, feeling flu-like and a whole series of other symptoms.

Music was and is a very important factor in my life. Nowadays I can no longer sing or play my guitar, because I have asthma, arthritis and other conditions. I do still have tapes, which make me very happy because when I listen to them, I can travel back in my thoughts to the time when I recorded them. Because I react to chemical substances, I cannot take any pain medication for the arthritis, so I use the music as a painkiller. My dear husband Mikael has placed a CD player next to my bed, so that during painful moments I can play the music which at that moment works as the best medicine (this changes each day and with each different mood). I lie on the bed with my eyes closed and go for a journey with the music: for me it really is a journey. One of my favorite "painkillers" is the music of Enya, an Irish singer who takes me to places far above the Earth. I change into a kind of cloud and "fly" away on it. Since my move to Fano I regularly undergo acupuncture treatments and this has made life a good deal better — but when I have lots of pain in between these treatments, I go with the "music therapy."

MCS has also had an enormous impact on my social life. Various friends have vanished into thin air. Half of my family members choose to smoke cigarettes and wear perfumed products instead of being able to visit me and I absolutely can't change this. All (!) MCS patients have encountered these kinds of situations.

I do not know any MCS patients who do not have trouble obtaining understanding from others, including the recognition that MCS is not a hysteria, but that we really do get sick — sometimes even for many days — after being exposed to something which we can't tolerate. I started my website because I wanted to share my knowledge with people who are looking for information and want to know more about MCS. I often say: "If I am able to somewhat help others with the knowledge gained during my painful fight for just welfare benefits, then it wasn't all for nothing and it had a purpose." My pain eases each time I am able to help others.

103. Moon McNeill, 50, Germany

Founder, international MCS artists' network, www.creativecanaries.org

When I was fourteen I had the first symptoms of an amalgam mercury poisoning. The symptoms varied from depression to insomnia, headaches, aggressiveness, a metal taste in my mouth and persistent dental problems. I absolutely did not understand what caused it. My health further deteriorated after a move to an apartment with a lot of processed wood, a synthetic carpet and anti-moth strips in the closet. My immune system began abandoning me every now and then. I had a constant pain in my muscles and bones and always felt ill. I was once such an energetic woman, but not much was left of that; I felt more like a seventy-year-old! In 1980 I began reacting to perfume, smoke, herbs, varnish, laundry detergents, et cetera.

But only in 2000, after I collapsed and was brought to a health clinic in Germany, did I realize thanks to the responses from the doctors that I strongly reacted to all kinds of chemicals even in low doses. This diagnosis brought about a turning point in my life. I was always active as an amateur artist, but my true passion, painting, remained unfulfilled. This became my goal, but with the diagnosis of MCS it became very difficult to find safe materials. It took me two years to discover that there are no safe materials for painting. The only challenge was to learn to handle the materials with wisdom and utmost carefulness. This required wearing masks, proper ventilation and taking other precautionary measures (above all, shutting out the dangerous materials).

Because of this quest, in 2001 I started an international network, Artists with MCS, in order to exchange ideas and advice with other artists experiencing the same problems. The network now has fifty members and has since changed its name: Creative Canaries. Discussing my artistic problems with other artists has done me lots of good. It has encouraged me to become the artist I always wanted to become — despite my chemical sensitivities.

Moon's art can be seen at: www.kun st.ag/Moon.McNeill

104. Silvia Müller, 43, Germany

Founder, Chemical Sensitivity Network (CSN), www.csn-deutschland. de

Creativity and the gift of using simple objects to produce works of art caused me to choose a trade in which I could use my skills. I finished my education as a decorator (interior design) in a warehouse. In the beginning my problems came in phases, usually accompanied by a serious headache and other symptoms that sometimes persisted for a long time, sometimes not. Sometimes I suddenly had teary eyes, would literally be seeing cross-eyed and had trouble with dizziness and bouts of lethargy. Sometimes I'd suddenly become very nauseous, which could last for hours before disappearing again for months. After a while I got chronic ailments, such as a loss of hearing, which kept getting worse. For years I did not consider it remotely possible that my ailments were related to my workplace. By coincidence I discovered one morning why my health and my colleagues' health was often so bad or even deteriorating: the cause of our problems was the harmful insecticides (organophosphates, lindan and pyrethroid) that in the evenings were misted or sprayed within the building, without the air being purified through the air conditioning system. I would arrive at work at six o'clock in the morning, but the air conditioning did not turn on until after eight o'clock, meaning that if they had sprayed again, I was in a very poisonous environment. Because cockroaches are hard to exterminate and the company was afraid the clients would discover the cockroaches, insecticides were sprayed regularly for twelve years. My colleagues also became sick, which was noticeable in the mood at work. Aggression and exhaustion often cropped up, which must also have been noticeable to the clients. We dragged ourselves through the days only to immediately go to bed once we got home. It became a race against time. I actually was completely

unaware of how dangerous and irreparable the damage caused by the poisoning was. It almost cost me my life. At a certain time my symptoms no longer improved on the weekends and I spent days sleeping. Added to that were also my ever-worsening respiratory problems and heart ailments. My tongue almost always lacked feeling and it was difficult for me to speak, as if it had been numbed. My own perfume gave me bad headaches and I also reacted more strongly to paint and varnish.

At a certain moment my health deteriorated very quickly and I broke down. Doctors still had no clue but they did see that I was very ill. The only way out was a treatment in the Environmental Health Center in Dallas with Dr. Rea. There they were able to ascertain serious damage to my immune and nervous systems. Tests also confirmed that I react strongly to various everyday chemical substances, numerous nutrients, molds, pollen, medicines, et cetera. Staying in the clinic was tough. There wasn't a single food item that I could endure without side effects. Many chemicals incited strong reactions and I often became unconscious. Many times I was hooked up to oxygen and an IV.

By then my whole family had changed their daily habits. From that moment on they only purchased organic products and only used chemical-free and perfume-free cleaning and care products. This also led to the creation of our family enterprise, Pure Nature (www.purenature.de). It began with a few products for ourselves and some fellow patients and grew into a company with over two thousand products and fourteen (part-time) employees, who incidentally are all themselves allergic or sensitive to chemicals. Pure Nature is not just a company; it is also a necessary project helping people adjust their lives.

At home, a special room was arranged to give me a possibility for betterment and some recovery. In my "survival room" only metal and glass were used and there is a hardwood floor. There are no books, no television, and the like. This room is still entirely intact and it also contains my oxygen machine, so that I can recover quickly in this space when something has made me sick. Due to diligent behavior (I had to stay inside for six years, often even wearing a mask) and the necessary support, I eventually reached such stability that nowadays I'm able to function somewhat in a safe environment. At home and in the car I use an air purifier, I use a water filter and I eat foods without additives, et cetera. Wherever I go, I need to know for certain ahead of time whether the space is suitable for me or not. Certain chemicals still cause serious symptoms and I can lose consciousness within one to two minutes if I don't leave a toxic area on time.

I have learned to accept this as a normal part of my life, just as I had to accept that I will never have a normal job, have children, or even spend a day like everyone else would. Life with MCS is an involuntarily hard and lonely life. Ever since my thirtieth birthday I have been declared 90 percent unable to work and have received a disability pension. I have concluded that there are many people in Germany with chemical sensitivity and that an upwards trend is at hand. The victims are left to themselves,

and if they can't find help from their relatives and friends, they are left to face their illness entirely alone. For this reason I founded the Chemical Sensitivity Network (CSN) ten years ago, and I use my remaining energy to help other people.

Recently I've married a dentist who has a lot of knowledge regarding medical establishments and also MCS. He completely adjusted his practice using air purifiers, safe (yet still disinfecting) cleaning products, et cetera. His colleagues have also been well served by these changes. One assistant no longer has headaches while another no longer suffers from asthma. Everyone feels better and happier in this healthier work environment, aside from the fact that it benefits productivity. A chemical-free environment isn't just good for MCS patients, but for us all!

I would like to say to everyone: "Stay positive, make sure you obtain the necessary knowledge about MCS, and dare to try new things, even if it takes just some small steps. Seize your chances and take responsibility by also helping others with your knowledge. Change your life and take on the challenge of MCS. You can definitely find improvement, but it requires sacrifices, sometimes large ones."

105. Gordon D. McHendry, 53, Scotland

Founder, MCS International: www. mcs-international.org

Mercury amalgam, crop spraying, and an ancient electrical fire extinguisher; these are some of my top suspects for kick-starting a decade and a half of increasingly severe Multiple Chemical Sensitivity (MCS), which was made many orders of magnitude worse when I innocently moved into a newly built bungalow. I then had to spend over five years sleeping every single night in my garden shed, all the year round and in all weathers. It is actually something of a minor miracle that I am still here to tell the tale today. The bottom line is this: I know about Multiple Chemical Sensitivity (MCS) — mild to severe — from long and very hard-won experience. I never asked for it, but I've had enough experiences with MCS to make me an expert!

The substances that make me sick are, among others: all perfumed personal care products, cleaning detergents (even many "natural" products), synthetic additives in food and drink, non-organic fruit and vegetables, solvents, paint, exhaust fumes, fire retardants, alcohol, et cetera. My MCS symptoms are, among others: lack of oxygen, irregular heartbeat, sleep apnea, fatigue, nightmares, short-term memory lapses, problems with concentration, brain fog, muscle spasms, speech problems, symptoms of poisoning (such as nausea), physical weakness, chronic skin rashes, shaking or shivering, restlessness or agitation, et cetera.

Before a worsening of both my MCS and my general cognitive abilities forced me to give it all up, I was a keen PC system builder. I managed to build over two dozen complete PC systems (and a handful of partial builds), and repair perhaps as many again, before I finally had to give it up. I really miss all that. It was a fascinating and exciting self-financing hobby and it was also excellent as a "keep-you-sane" therapy against the life-stealing isolation imposed on you by the very disabling combination of severe MCS and ME/CFS. These days I live alone, divorced, and have a 27-year-old son. Due to MCS I try to prevent people from visiting me as much as possible and when I travel, I always do so protected by a mask and a small air purification system.

For more information on my personal struggle with MCS, you can also see my personal website: www.satori-5.co.uk/ 2_mcs/2_fpe/2_fpe.html. I founded MCS International in order to bring to light the hidden dangers of modern synthetic chemicals — globally! I could very much use help from volunteers from all nations in this effort! So become a member and help us in this good cause. You yourself decide how much time to devote and what you would mean for the project.

106. Christian Schifferle, 52, Switzerland

Founder, Swiss MCS association: www.mcs-liga.ch

At the time I became seriously ill, I was living in Zurich in a shared apartment building where a number of people lived and shared a communal living room. I had come to the city to escape the agricultural poisons, which by then already made me sick. In that regard the city seemed cleaner than the countryside, but in the city I came to deal with neighbors who often used substances I couldn't tolerate. And how do you make clear to your neighbors and housemates that they should stop using these substances? Below me lived a chain smoker who frequently sprayed all sorts of air fresheners in her room to cover the smell of smoke. All around the house hung perfume vapors. From all the rooms wafted laundry detergent and perfume scents. Not for a second did I have clean air anymore. In the living room lay a hardwood floor that had been varnished. On a hot summer's day, when my attic room was terribly hot again and the perfume vapors caused severe symptoms, I fled to a camping ground where I lived in my car for a year. Now I spend the entire year in an RV, in which I keep the TV and computer behind glass, because the fumes and radiation from these devices make me sick. There is no running water in the RV and I can't make use of the bathroom buildings because they contain too many chemical substances, such as cleaning detergents, perfume and disinfecting substances.

When I am exposed to chemical substances, I get serious symptoms, as if my whole body has fallen into poison oak. The heavier the substances, the more severe my reactions. My lungs hurt, I get cramps and spasms in my body and all my mucous membranes swell up.

It's as if I'm afflicted with a chronic flu. On the good days it's like a normal cold and on the bad days I feel like I've got a fever of 104 degrees. If I've inhaled, for example, solvent vapors or hair spray, I get trouble with speech and concentration, I begin to stutter and I simply can't find the right words. Besides MCS I also have CFS and fibromyalgia. During the high season in the summer and winter many tourists come to the campground and I unfortunately have to flee from there as well; I then take my car into the forests and sleep in a reclining chair in the open air. I'm always relieved when I've endured another winter at the campground, because it's not always easy. Last year I had a lung infection and wasn't able to take anything for it because I can't tolerate medicine. Severely ill, I had to brave the freezing cold just to get water.

From my trailer I run the Swiss MCS association, which three hundred people have now joined. But this is just the tip of the iceberg. We are trying hard to get this disease finally recognized. As of today MCS is still considered a mental illness in Switzerland and because of this it's extremely difficult to receive understanding and sympathy from your family and relatives. It's also very difficult to pay for the costs incurred due to MCS on the very low disability benefits. For example, we can barely afford an expensive air purifier, even though we really need one to clean the air. The fact that you have to spend every day living like an outcast, without any form of companionship as if you're on another planet, is of course entirely outlandish. This environmental illness is without question an alarm call by nature.

11

The Voices of MCS Patients from the Netherlands

107. Jolanda, 43

For over ten years I worked for a company producing laundry and cleaning products, in their marketing department. I was primarily engaged with product development, meaning I often was exposed to perfumes and synthetic substances. My MCS-related ailments really started coming through when all kinds of liquid toilet products and air fresheners started hitting the market. These ailments worsened when we moved into a new building. I personally think that a combination of factors kept making me more sensitive.

I often had a shortness of breath and began reacting to cigarette smoke, solvents and various perfumed products. For a long time I was very tired. I noticed that new chemicals kept adding to the list of those to which I reacted, sometimes quite severely. I suffered from swollen sinuses (which sometimes gave me such bad headaches that I would have to stay in bed for a few days), sinus infections (for which I had surgery), et cetera. By avoiding the substances that make me sick and by adhering to a diet, I now no longer have these problems. Now, when I do get exposed to substances harmful to me, my symptoms are: a tingling sensation in my tongue, pangs of pain in my jaw and neck, nausea, general malaise, et cetera. The fol-lowing day I'm extremely tired and I often have itchy or tired eyes. I now realize it much faster when something is wrong and am more able to take measures on time. My life has changed because of chemical sensitivity, but due to the adjustments I made, things are going well.

The following changes, among others, are very important for me: consistent avoidance of synthetic substances, eating organic food and not eating foods to which I don't react well. I like to undergo bioresonance therapy, and I regularly get a foot reflexology massage, which relaxes me and does me a great deal of good. My work has changed and I now work from home, which is a very good solution. I do everything to make sure I can keep doing so. I'm lucky to have many people near me who are very respectful of me and help me out. My family and friends have adapted themselves very well and always are considerate of me, which I think is wonderful. You do sometimes hear less fortunate stories.

I myself also went through a very difficult time, before everything in my life adjusted so well. But I would not have wanted it any other way, because this hardship has spiritually enriched me and allowed me to grow within. I found my inner strength and was therefore able to assume a more vulnerable and soft disposition. I have become a better person and I think that handicaps and setbacks could usually do this for a person, if only the person sets out to handle problems in a positive way. Thanks to my experiences I now get more enjoyment from the small things, especially the things which I no longer take for granted. Despite the circumstances, I have a found a manner of living in which I can function well, and with this I am at peace.

108. Anonymous, 56

For almost five years I have been sick and at home. How it all started is difficult to retrace, because various issues contributed. Different events and critical situations have taken place in my life. After a very drastic incident I was sick for a while and suffered infections, especially in my muscles and tendons. I also had a great deal of pain in my back. After doing some tests, my doctor diagnosed me with fibromyalgia, and these ailments have never really gone away. Sometimes they're less present and sometimes they're worse. During that time I also became allergic or sensitive to many chemical substances. Almost everything was unbearable on my skin. I could only endure silk. After a few years my allergies became less severe and I was still able to combine my family and my work, despite the fibromyalgia.

In the past I used to work in advertising and I used a lot of solvents. Later on, when I was working in a hospital, a fire broke out and I inhaled poisonous fumes. As a result I got problems with my lungs and often was short of breath.

A number of years later I underwent a serious operation and since then I've never really recovered. My employer moved to a new office with an entirely new inventory and a closed air conditioning system, and my ailments kept getting worse. It began with coughing, skin problems and severe exhaustion. After that I twice went into anaphylactic shock and in between also had bouts of Ménière's disease, which is an illness resulting in attacks of dizziness, tinnitus and a loss of hearing. Because of this and my reaction to personal care products (such as hair gel and makeup) and the perfume scents people carry on them, I can no longer go to work. In the psychiatry department where I worked at the time, patients are allowed to smoke in certain areas, which made it impossible for me to be there. After extensive testing by an allergist at a university hospital, I was diagnosed with asthma. At the same time it was determined that I react sensitively to certain substances in the air, which I inhale and which I exposed to via my skin.

When I am exposed to chemical substances such as perfume or solvents, my symptoms are: severe (allergic) reactions, such as skin rashes, shortness of breath, pain in my whole body, the feeling that something is fizzing just below my skin, headaches, emotionality, joint pains, intestinal problems, frequent coughing, poor vision, chronic fatigue and general malaise. In short, I felt very, very ill. I underwent various tests with an internist, an allergist, a dermatologist, an ear, nose and throat specialist, a psychiatrist and a neurologist, but nobody could help me and I did not get well. Now I'm undergoing treatment by an anthroposophical doctor and, with many adjustments, my life has become bearable.

Using an air purifier, I make sure my home constantly has clean air, and because of this things aren't as bad as they once were. I'm doing pretty well. I pay close attention to my diet, lead a regular life, and I make sure to relax and get some physical exercise, by going on walks, for example. Yet my life has completely changed. I can no longer work, people can no longer pop in to visit, I can't go anywhere just on a whim (due to perfume and laundry products, among other things), my house can't be painted, I'm unable to perform my own household chores and due to the respiratory problems my energy level is very limited. I am severely disabled.

109. Julia Slenders, 60

For sixteen years now I have been a bedridden chronic fatigue syndrome (CFS) patient with rheumatism, and for this I need home care, help and assistance. By repeatedly getting exposed to, among other things, the perfume of a care provider, I furthermore developed MCS. Because this person came to help me multiple times per week, I kept getting exposed to it and kept getting sicker and more sensitive. Of course I tried getting perfume-free help but this turned out to be very difficult or, in fact, impossible. With other general aid services it was also not possible to receive perfume-free care or assistance. I have noticed that these kinds of agencies don't want to cooperate, because this "would encroach on the private rights of the employees." Presumably they didn't even ask if anyone with the organization would be willing to do this for me. The decision in this regard is apparently dependent on what the staff or management personally thinks of the situation.

In this way I'm excluded from care, in the wealthy Netherlands which is supposed to have a good social security system. I have a right to help, but nobody arranges anything for me. I'm left completely to my own fate, all because I'm a victim of generally accepted "right" to "smell nice." It's seen as my problem, which they want nothing to do with. Due to my chemical sensitivity I can't make use of a home food service because of all the synthetic additives in the food. I can't ride along with medical transports and effectively have to do without an eye doctor, dietician, speech therapist, et cetera. Fortunately I have a perfume-free general practitioner who comes and takes blood samples at my home, because the diagnostic center refuses to eliminate perfumes. It took me seven years to find perfume-free psychiatric help and a physiotherapist who would accommodate my needs. If somebody walks in wearing perfume, my whole body goes haywire and it takes days for me to recover. In these cases my chronic fatigue symptoms also acutely worsen. Within my home I have adjusted everything I need, such as laundry and cleaning products and scent-free care products.

This situation, especially the social exclusion — which I experience as extremely difficult and inhumane — is very hard to bear! It's incredibly tiring and taxing to always be asking for care.

Again and again you have to deal with rejections, even though I'm dependent on others, so I have to keep ringing the bell. This has become a desperate situation which exacts its toll on me, causes me great sadness and above all suffocates me with loneliness.

110. Margot, 49

Until my eighteenth birthday I was a healthy person with a zest for life, a real go-doer. Except for some allergies to dust mites and animals, there really wasn't anything wrong with me. I enjoyed life and everything it offered. When I was eighteen I received a few heavy anesthetics, and after that the first serious ailments began, such as a loss of concentration and severe exhaustion. When I was twenty I had mononucleosis and six months later I developed various food allergies. First I was only allergic to alcohol and spices, but later also to many other foods. Over time new problems kept coming. I had muscle and joint pains, intestinal problems, balance disorders, a chronic flu-like feeling, frequent headaches, and I was often nauseous.

The doctors had no answer for my symptoms. I was eventually no longer able to tolerate the medicines that were prescribed for me—I had apparently become sensitive to medicine. I missed work on several occasions for long periods and eventually, when I was thirty-two, I was diagnosed with CFS and declared partially unfit for work.

I heard of MCS for the first time five years ago. Looking back, I can see I have had recognizable ailments related to chemical substances since I was eighteen (since the anesthesia). It became very clear after I'd done a lot of painting in our home, after which I got sick if I even just smelled paint.

As a result of my chemical sensitivities we had to take many measures in our home towards avoiding chemicals as much as possible. We only used natural paint products, but even these I myself can no longer use. Our furniture, floor covering and bedding was all adjusted, and I also replaced all cleaning products, skin care products, cosmetics and laundry products with natural products that do not contain perfume or essential oils. Unfortunately I also developed electro-sensitivity, which necessitated even more adjustments to, among others, the telephone and the computer.

I kept coming home from work sick (nausea and headaches), until I figured out that it was caused by the air fresheners at work. This made me even more sensitive, especially to perfumes and laundry products on other people's clothing, but unfortunately also to other products, such as plastic, rubber, printing ink, emission fumes, and wood stoves.

In a short period this has turned my life completely upside down; it causes tons of limitations and puts me in considerable isolation. I can no longer go to public establishments, going to work is no longer an option, shopping for groceries is a serious hassle and birthday parties are impossible to visit for me. When people want to come visit me, they have to wash their clothes using perfume-free laundry products and not wear any perfume or other scent at all. A number of friends have dropped out because of this. It's asking too much of them to maintain contact given such a strict protocol, aside from the fact that of course it's all become very one-sided, as I can never go visit them. Luckily, my family tries its very best and that is a welcome source of support because such assistance is highly needed in these situations. But above all it's an enormous blessing that I have such a wonderful partner who supports me immensely.

Our recently renovated home is now giving me problems once again. The neighbor's laundry, the cars in the street — everything weighs heavily on me these days. Our house has been sealed on the inside and outside as much as possible and we're able to keep the ground floor clean with two air purifiers. Because of the increased ailments associated with electro smog, living inside our home has gotten even more complex. For over half a year now I have primarily lived in the kitchen, where at night I also lay out my bed. We'll be forced to move to a freestanding home, far from neighbors. At our new place I'd like to try to remedy the lack of social contacts. I want to make a reception space with a glass wall and an intercom. This will be a kind of closed veranda, hermetically sealed from my living quarters. My visitors can sit on one side of the glass wall and I on the other. In this way I won't get sick from chemical substances but will still have a way of meeting people. I will be able to welcome people who just want to drop by, even if they weren't able to properly prepare for the visit. Life is no longer easy, but I plan to make the best of it.

111. Dick Prasing, 70

By living in a house for twenty years in which many materials were processed and chemicals like formaldehyde were gassing out, I developed MCS. After spending a night in the attic, which contained lots of particle board, I got the first symptoms, such as edema in my face. Because of constant exposures I slowly got more sensitive and more ill; I also started getting depressed and had thoughts about ending my own life, because at the time I no longer saw any possible way to make something of my life.

The poisoning had made my life very difficult; it limited me in my freedom and my social contacts became complicated as well. Nobody understood that I could get so sick from chemical substances. I reacted very sensitively to smoke, perfume, and laundry products. On top of it all, I also became very sensitive to food products and medicines. A neurologist put me in touch with Mr. Kamsteeg of the Centre for Environmental Medicine (www.keac.nl), who in turn connected me with Dr. Rea. Because of this I started reading about MCS a lot and completely recognized my situation in the literature. I got in touch with the Dutch Patients and Consumers Platform and informed them of my situation. They had never heard of MCS, but they did write down my name, allowing other people with the same problems to get in touch with me. From this the MCS Self Help Group arose, because there was a demand for a support group wherein people could exchange experiences, information and tips with one another. After all, together we know more than a single person does. We were able to help each other in all kinds of areas. In the end I no longer had enough energy to lead this group and I'm therefore very grateful to my successor for taking over for me.

After living in an urban area for twenty years we moved to the countryside where the air is quite a bit cleaner, making it easier for me to be outside, although, in my current place of residence, my sensitivity is once again increasing due to agriculture and spraying with pesticides and weed killers. The wind blows these substances all throughout the area. And unfortunately social contacts aren't easy here either, because of my situation and a lack of understanding.

I recently became a member of a lawn bowling club so I can enjoy the outside, although I have to be careful not to get too close to people using perfumed products. In this way I try to do have some fun while still avoiding chemical substances as much as possible. I can no longer attend church due to the laundry product scents and the like used by fellow churchgoers, and I'm thus forced to follow the church services through the online radio. I also still can't entertain visitors, and even then I can only see people who have somewhat adjusted themselves. When visitors yet again bring with them too much scent and chemical substances, it all goes terribly wrong and I go upstairs, sick and in tears.

112. Anonymous, 57

About eighteen years ago I was walking through the town in which I lived, next to an orchard where right that moment somebody was busy spraying the trees with insecticide. Because the wind was blowing in my direction, I was covered with a full load and I therefore also inhaled it. Besides the fact that this was a very unpleasant experience, I had no idea at the time what long-term consequences were in store for me. It happened around the same time as when I was doing lots of chores and projects around the house as well. When something had to be painted, I'd be the one to do it. Whether the walls had to be painted or the hardwood floor had to be varnished, I'd take care of it.

After these experiences my body slowly began reacting more sensitively to substances that previously had been no problem at all! If I breathed in tobacco smoke, for example, I would get considerable respiratory problems, and I also got all kinds of symptoms when exposed to perfume, aftershave, air fresheners, laundry products, fireplaces, ink, and vehicle traffic. And over time it just kept getting worse! My primary symptoms are: headaches, itchy eyes, pain in my ears, swollen glands and mucous membranes, speech difficulties, heart palpitations, cold sweats, dizziness, extreme exhaustion and painful joints. After reading a Dutch newspaper article about MCS, I discovered that apparently my ailments had a name! I then found more information about MCS and began making changes, of which avoiding the substances that make sick is the most important.

Fortunately, I can still work because I have a glass room at my workplace, giving me good protection from my (scented) colleagues. Of course it's not always possible to avoid everything and I am frequently still exposed to all kinds of irritants from aftershaves and perfumes. At work I always use the bathroom for disabled persons, where the air freshener has been removed, and I take the elevator meant for goods, in order to avoid my colleagues as much as possible.

For about a year now I have also regularly had stomach and intestinal problems, which when they arise put me on non-active status for up to a week, to my great dismay. But I discovered that eating organic foods is the silver bullet. My symptoms have strongly receded and I can keep on going, much improved. New things keep cropping up and sometimes it's a real struggle to live and work with MCS. Fortunately it hasn't yet driven me into isolation, like you sometimes hear about from others. But it does make me very sick all too often.

113. Marianne, 48

As a child I was already bothered by the heavy cigar and cigarette smoke that always hung in the air. I'd get a sore throat, headaches and would sniffle for days. Once I started living on my own I developed allergies to cats and dust mites. I was also diagnosed with asthma. Over the years I kept getting more sensitive to cigarette smoke and when I went to a place where people were smoking, my eyes, throat and head would hurt and I'd usually feel very ill the next day.

In 1994 a brain tumor was discovered in my youngest son. A long period of treatments followed and I was often with him in the hospital, where I was always very short of breath. I'm sad to say he died two years ago. At the time I considered it totally normal that I'd be short of breath, given all the emotions coursing through my body.

After I had refurnished all the rooms in the house — painting, wallpapering, moving furniture et cetera — I had awful headaches and was intensely tired. I again thought that my ailments were caused by the death of my son and paid them no attention. Later my husband and I moved to a new apartment and again I did a lot of painting. I also treated the ceiling in the bathroom with some chemical designed to prevent mold. We had purchased new furniture and curtains and had new floor covering put in. The combination of all the new items, the painting, and the polluted air inside the building in which I worked (the air vents were all completely blackened) at the time probably made me very sick. The occupational therapist said it was a burn-out but, looking back, I had the same symptoms then as I do now.

It took a whole year before I was able to return to work full time. When I started work in a new building, I noticed that slowly things were getting worse with me and that I'd begun reacting to all kinds of chemical substances, including my own perfume, which from then on I never used again. I also started having trouble with electro smog. The filters on the air conditioning in that building hadn't been replaced for years, which may have caused my migraines and further worsened my MCS. But I didn't realize that then. My colleagues and other people in the building also had various maladies, such as dry eyes and sinus infections. Eventually my symptoms got so bad I could no longer work at all, while blood tests revealed nothing.

My symptoms are: heart palpitations, headaches, chronic fatigue, sensitivity to light and sound, sore throat, shortness of breath, stomach and intestinal problems, mood swings, difficulties with concentration and short-term memory, muscle and joint pains, poor sleep, night sweats and so on. Since I made various adjustments, including the avoidance of perfumed care products, things are going a little better with me. But I do unfortunately keep coming across new things I can't tolerate, which I then have to add to the list of things I have avoid.

114. Annelies, 54

In January 2006, after repeated exposures to a combination of substances, such as hyacinths sprayed with pesticides, construction materials and chemical cleaning products in a nursing home, I started getting irritated mucous membranes and other ailments. My sense of smell had always been quite sharp, but was now excessively strong and I began reacting to ever more chemical substances with burning and painful mucous membranes (eyes, nose, throat and lips), headaches, dizziness and heart palpitations. Before my exposures in the nursing home, I already had all kinds of vague difficulties with my health — too many to mention — and already had an aversion to certain substances (incense, heavy perfumes and fireworks), but I

did not notice direct detrimental effects upon my well-being. During visits to a garden center I often struggled with sudden spells of dizziness and muscle weakness in my legs, or later in the day got a strong migraine, but I never made the connection to the chemical substances found at the garden center and attributed it to other causes. The relationship between my ailments and chemicals in the environment only became clear to me many years down the road.

After looking for information on my by then intense reactions to almost all synthetic scents, I found a name for this phenomenon: MCS. It was now clear to me: for years, without knowing it, I'd been sick due to an environment that is unhealthy for me. From experience I already knew that I was sensitive to items such as food preservatives, coloring substances, taste strengtheners, certain medications and heavy metals such as mercury in amalgams. I avoid those items as much as possible. It's hard, but doable. The recently developed perfume intolerance does make life far more complex. Even in the outside air these scents often blow all around me.

Because of my health condition I could no longer work and therefore, as well as the lack of understanding on the part of various people around me, my world became quite small. A few good — apparently real — friends kept coming. In time, going on vacations became too taxing, but I did not live in isolation: I could, when I felt well enough (the severity of the symptoms was variable), still do lots of things with friends, such as shopping, going out to eat, take relaxing courses and make short trips. And furthermore I did and do know how to keep myself busy and I developed new interests, so I didn't disappear in a "black hole." But due to my chemical sensitivity the little bit of social life that I do still have has changed drastically: I'm largely penned to my home, where everything that has scents or is synthetic has as much as possible been removed. Receiving guests is problematic, because no matter how sympathetically they try to be chemical- and scent-free, it's an almost impossible task for them — especially if they travel using public transportation where they of course absorb all sorts of substances from perfumes on other people. I myself also can no longer travel using public transportation, which makes my world smaller than it already was.

115. Anonymous, 38

Though I'm a sporty girl and come from an even sportier family, I've had allergies since my early youth. As a child the fumes from glue made me nauseous. Once, during volleyball practice, I was suddenly covered in welts. My head, hands and one foot grew swollen out of proportion. I became hoarse, could barely breathe, and was weak and listless. Various tests at the hospital showed that I had strong allergic reactions to a number of substances in food and in the air. Apparently I had a life-threatening allergy. Due to my anaphylaxis, from then on I always had to carry an adrenaline injection.

At the Art Academy I had to work with wood glue and treated wood that made me sick. If material from the pre-

vious class was hardening in the classroom, I couldn't sit through the period due to headaches, disorientation and nausea. I'd have to open the window or come back at a later hour to make up the practical section of class.

After two years at the Art Academy I became pregnant and decided to get a job at a printing press, because I was going to become a single parent. The smell of the fresh printing ink often was too much for me, but I figured pregnant women often were bothered by certain smells. After my son was born, I decided to reduce my work in the press to just one day a week, while doing work for the company at home.

I was asked to make the décor for an annual party. Because it had to be visible from the very back of the room, I decided to outline it with marker. The décor was almost finished when I suddenly got an awful headache. I also became nauseous, shaky and disoriented, a condition which lasted a few days.

Things like gatherings in public spaces, riding in a car and basking in the pool no longer went well for me, causing symptoms like a swollen throat, headache, nauseous, disorientation and a wheezy cough. Using a Ménière test, the ear, nose and throat specialist determined that my balance was teetering on the edge of the allowable limit, and I was prescribed medicine for balance disorders.

As a single parent with household chores and work to do, fatigue was not exactly something I could give in to. An internal specialist determined I had a "heavily neglected case of mono." A "strange protein" was found in my blood. Perhaps I could recognize in myself the condition chronic fatigue syndrome?

I kept getting more pains and was referred to a rheumatologist, who diagnosed me with fibromyalgia. After I met my current husband and married him, we moved to our new house. The wooden floor was varnished by my husband. It must have been heavy stuff, because it made me quite "high." For months after the move I was miserable. I could no longer stay in drugstores, shoe stores, sporting goods stores or jeans stores for extended periods. I kept thinking it just wasn't my day, but the incidents kept on coming. If I put on nail polish it was like I'd been slapped in the face, and I'd get "high" at the hair salon. Working as a house cleaner, which I'd done for years, was no longer possible and I ended up finding other work.

One time I was staining the fence in our yard, as well as painting the roof of the bike shed. I had to do it little by little, because I realized I couldn't do work like that for long periods at a time. While doing this work I suddenly felt an enormous headache and nausea come up and I collapsed. My body went completely limp and I was gasping for air. Our doctor was off duty, but a different doctor said it was an allergic reaction to the paint. Pale as a ghost, I lay on the couch shaking for hours.

I started reacting to everything: glue, paint, perfumes, laundry detergents and fabric softeners, smoke, car exhaust, newspapers. This sensitivity made it very difficult for me to go to a supermarket or shopping mall. At a hospital I became disoriented from the cleaning and disinfecting products. I became ill

at a shoe store. I once collapsed in the changing room of a clothing store. My skin gave me more and more problems and appeared to be a "pollution meter" in terms of its itchiness. My sense of smell also seemed to increase strongly. The general practitioner mentioned something about a rosacea and established the presence of an infection in my blood. He prescribed a course of antibiotics for two months which turned out to be ineffective. The burning sensation on my skin persisted and worsened in polluted environments. I could only endure the sun when wearing very high protection factor sun block, but there were few to no sunscreen products that didn't make me "high."

My health was falling apart. After eleven years of volunteer work for various associations, I felt it was necessary to quit doing that as well. I myself no longer used perfumed products, but I soon had to ask my husband and child to do the same. Due to my rheumatism and pelvic instability (PGP) I became tied to the home and was thus unable to do practically anything. I was assigned home care. With endless therapeutic exercises we have been able to slowly build everything up again. It was a complete rehabilitation process, wherein my family and friends supported us — for which we are very grateful!

At the allergist we discovered I also had asthma and with proper medication we were able to control that as well. We sanitized our home and, following the advice of a lung specialist, we paid even greater attention to minimizing chemical substances. Little by little my tolerance increased. As a result, we as a family have had to forgo a great deal of spontaneity and freedom of movement. Many things are still an attack on my body, even when on the surface you often can't tell.

116. Dick van Nieuwkoop, 51

On a lovely summer's day, when I was just six months old, my mother laid me down on the grass in the yard. A short while later I spent six months in the hospital with a very serious form of eczema (neurodermatitis). It was so bad they placed my arms in tubes so I could no longer scratch them. It turned out I was very allergic to grass and tree pollen, cats and all kinds of food products. I also developed asthma.

As a young adult I lived in a town called Lisse, where among other things small airplanes sprayed pesticides on the farmlands. Many years later I had a small sound studio there. At that time I spent also some time in New York and Los Angeles, where I had some serious health ailments which I then did not fully understand. For my studio work I moved to Hilversum, where my asthma disappeared like snow under a hot sun. When I went to visit my mother in Lisse, the asthma often returned immediately. In Hilversum I lived and worked in a street with little traffic. But slowly the street got busier and I started feeling less well. I also had problems with my eyes and back, problems with concentration and memory lapses. Then several road changes in town made my street one of the busiest, and from that moment on I could barely get out of bed

from exhaustion. At that time I also got a wound on my head that just wouldn't heal. I then began experimenting with air purifiers and water vaporizers, and thanks to the results I was fortunately able to continue my work. When I was on vacation I noticed that in places without traffic or industrial areas, my eczema always disappeared. In Israel and Indonesia, for example, things went better for me and in Thailand even the wound on my head healed.

In 1991 I moved to the peaceful town of Almere because I felt so much better there. There I built a new place with two studios and a modern air treatment system. Unfortunately the town grew at a very rapid pace, causing the traffic and the exhaust from the town heating center to increase, as well as the number of flights from Schiphol airport passing over Almere. Added to this was the fact that I lived in a new house with new construction materials, which gassed out all sorts of fumes. Eventually this caused an itch so bad that I had to sleep in the bathtub, with only my head above water, in order to spare my skin from exposure to the gases in the polluted air. I eventually lost my business because I was much too sick to work. I then moved to an outskirt of the town and experimented with a tent over my bed, outfitted with air purifiers and increased air pressure. I was also able to create a much higher humidity in the tent, which was good for my skin. With this I made some progress.

Together with a fellow patient I left for Vancouver Island, Canada, for three months in the summer of 2004. Staying in the relatively clean air did me a lot of good: among other things, my vision strongly improved, from 50 percent in the Netherlands to 80 percent in Canada. Yet shortly after returning to the Netherlands I was once again very ill. At that moment another MCS patient pointed me towards the IQAir Multigas air purifier. With this device inside a small tent I made good progress. But the result was that I almost never left the tent, because outside of it I'd soon get sick again. This air purifier removes a broad spectrum of gases — to which my father was also exposed during his entire life — from the air, while itself producing little to no gases, like some other air purifiers do. My father was a house painter and died from chronic toxic encephalopathy (CTE or psycho-organic syndrome). Even my grandfather, who was a bricklayer, had problems with eczema. In a newspaper article I discovered that the children of painters apparently have five to six times as many disorders as do the children of carpenters.

Using online satellite maps of air pollution, I went looking for the cleanest places on Earth for a new place to live. It would have to be New Zealand, South America, South Africa or Thailand. I still remembered my experience with the chronic head wound and I therefore decided in August 2005 to move to Thailand with the same woman I visited Canada with, who also had an increasingly severe case of MCS. After a month in Thailand the chronic wound had healed again and I decided to stay there to live. Today, about a year and a half later, you can only see a scar where the wound once was and my eczema has disappeared. I alternate between living in the city or in countryside in the far northeast of Thailand, depending on the burning of the rice fields and on the wet season. There is still no industrial development at all and barely any traffic, and I hope it stays that way. I'm often tired but usually not sick, and my brain is starting to function again. Here I am never itchy and my allergies have totally gone. It feels as if I won my life back. Due to the increasing air pollution in the Netherlands I'm unfortunately forced to live in exile.

Also see my website: www.xs4all.nl/~dvannieu/MCS/MCS.html

117. Mirjam Ruijter, 60

My father was an artist/painter with a studio in the home, in which I even slept for some time. There was thus often, besides the urban pollution, also a chemical exposure, from solvents, formalin and also cigarette smoke. After moving to a building near a car body shop, which leaked fumes from spray paint jobs, the living environment worsened even more. In the winters there were gases from the petrol stoves inside the house, some of which did not have an exhaust pipe. Because of this situation I often had headaches. From puberty onwards I had chronic laryngitis and often a burning pain when I went to the bathroom. I myself also became a sculptor and a graphic designer specializing in wood engraving, and though I had problems, I kept working in my studio among other artists who used solvents in copious amounts. In 1986 I painted a floor (wearing a gas mask) with a two-component polyurethane varnish with isocyanates (which was later prohibited for indoor use), which caused, among other things, three months of respiratory problems, an infection in my lung passages and possibly a preliminary phase of cancer and/or celiac disease. Because I kept doing the things I wanted and even felt I had to do, I developed CFS in 1989, while also increasing my sensitivity to all kinds of chemicals. In the warm months of 2003, I could barely move due to breathing problems. The doctors could not diagnose it: my lungs were in perfect condition. Even provocations using histamines did not incite a reaction. Later I read that the German toxicologist Daunderer and the American doctor Cheney explained this symptom as a lack of oxygen in the tissue and cells.

In 2004 I purchased a portable air filter with a head cover and, together with my fellow sufferer Dick, who in 2003 also had persistent ailments, spent three months on Vancouver Island, Canada, for its clean air. But by living in a house which was very moldy, contained pesticides and synthetic material and was also close to a road and a gas station, my symptoms actually worsened. Since then, in the Netherlands, I constantly have to protect myself with air purifiers. During an extended stay in Thailand over the following years, I was usually able to go without my mobile breathing protection device, as long as I was far enough away from car exhaust and other irritating substances. I also discovered that, if I hadn't been exposed to certain substances for a while, I'd be able to somewhat endure them again. Unfortunately Thailand is a "hot spot," meaning there is always the influence of smoke, which manifested, among other

things, in chronic exhaustion, often a feeling of drunkenness, pain when doing and repeating muscle exercises, and joint and skin problems. And because Dick and I were also together in Thailand, we would — just as in the Netherlands or Canada — both feel it at the same time if the air quality had worsened. We also noticed that the polluted air not only affected us but also others, who would then, just like us, feel ill for some time.

Since my return to Amsterdam I constantly protect myself, which has resulted in the near disappearance of the ailments I had in Thailand and, after a short while, the regular return of the pains that are typical for me in the Netherlands: pain in my intestines, bladder and mouth. Where I live, my protective measures often fail. This happens at times of air traffic over the city but also especially when the wind is coming from the northwest, dragging with it the polluted air from an industrial area. Or, for example, it happens when the neighbors take a shower, use care products on themselves or do the laundry. The perfume scents that arise from the products used in these activities first give me burning, itchy skin, then hot flashes, and then I feel miserable for a while.

My plan is to spend at least the warmer half of each year in a country with cleaner air, in a spot where I can usually be without having to wear my helmet. I hope that in time the air quality in the most polluted areas will improve, so that I eventually will no longer have to flee and that due to the cleaner air, less people will get sick.

Also see my blog: http://mirjam-gone-bananas-english.blogspot.com/

118. Anonymous, 57

In January 2005 I suddenly noticed that I reacted to the perfume in my laundry detergent with a painful, dry feeling in my eyes, especially the inner corners. This was the beginning of my MCS. In the following weeks I tried to avoid perfumes as much as possible and got in touch with fellow patients through a self help group for MCS patients. My MCS was then still in a mild phase. That changed, unfortunately, when I bought a car in April 2005, which was delivered after having been treated with "cockpit spray." Various attempts have been made at removing this substance, among other things by using a so-called professional cleaning product, which was not available in stores. Especially after inhaling this product I noticed a sudden deterioration. After this incident my sense of smell became stronger and I began reacting to a number of things. I have had various symptoms when I was exposed to perfume, dust, preservatives, synthetic color, scent and taste additives, phosphates, pesticides, insecticides, mold, car exhaust, printing ink, tobacco smoke, wood fires, gasoline, formaldehyde, rubber, pets, birds, plants and trees, ozone, electromagnetic radiation and geopathic zones, which emit low level gamma radiation.

My symptoms were painful eyes, numbness in my bottom lip, shortness of breath and weight loss. When I also became sensitive to my mattress and could no longer wear my clothes, the situation became unlivable. In July 2005, it turned out from testing that I also had a serious intolerance to pesticides on food and to various food products.

Since then I've only been eating organic food and I avoid certain foods, so some improvement has been made. I can once again go to stores without problems and receive guests. I do try persuading people to come over as scentless as possible. In the beginning this caused some problems, but fortunately most family members and friends have been prepared to be considerate of me in that regard.

It was an advantage that at the depth of my crisis I was living alone and did not have a job outside of the home. In that case the problems could have been much larger. My life has changed since MCS; I now live much more conscientiously and carefully. There may be some limitations — for example, I still can't go on vacation — but I'm not faced with serious isolation. I once again have hope for the future.

119. Willem Schneider, 73

First of all I ought to say I don't have it quite as a bad as some other MCS patients, which is why I call myself an "upcoming MCS patient." I'd like to tell my story to show that a person can suffer from certain chemical sensitivities without being a severe MCS patient. I think there are many people who lead a "normal" life but nonetheless react sensitively to certain substances, such as cigarette smoke (shortness of breath, headaches, clogged nose, et cetera). They also might have trouble (headaches, dizziness) when, for example, something was recently painted. How many people must there be who have migraines, sensitive airways, and the like, who often just aren't able to establish the link to their sensitivities to certain chemical substances? There are stories of people who had headaches for years and then switched to a different deodorant or stopped using their perfume for a period of time, and suddenly got rid of their chronic headache! How many people might there be who have headaches caused by the perfume they wear or from being stuck in traffic, who think they got the headache from the stress in their busy lives? The solution could be so simple!

I too was someone who didn't understand the source of such problems, which I usually had while on the road. You see, for years I was a representative, doing a lot of bumper-to-bumper driving. Of course, at the time I knew nothing of the harmful effects of driving right behind other cars. Sometimes I stepped out of my car feeling completely nauseous, but I still didn't realize that driving like this was harmful to my health. I had, however, already been staying as far away from perfume stores or hair salons as I could, because they smelled so strongly. It must have been halfway through the period during which I drove all around the Netherlands for work that I'd get sick from diesel cars when I had a cold. Coming home, I often hopped on my bike in order to clear my lungs, far from all the traffic. At the time I was still a smoker, which I immediately stopped upon seeing a public service advertisement announcing that if you smoked while driving, you were asking for heart problems. I then spent years fighting, along with my children, against my first wife's smoking habit.

Now I can no longer handle smoky air, which momentarily makes me hoarse. I also can't handle the smell of paint that contains solvents, but this I can live with. As I said, I'm lucky and am not as sick as many other people with chemical sensitivities. But I am happy to help create awareness of Multiple Chemical Sensitivity, because I am convinced that the cause of many problems can be found on that level.

120. Annie Terpstra, 47

I am a married mother of two children. We live in the northern part of the Netherlands, where there happens to be not much industry, meaning MCS is presumably not as common here. But alas, it did not prevent my developing MCS. About ten years ago my ailments started, probably because we lived right next door to a dry cleaner. My ailments were not really typical of MCS. It was just like hay fever: red eyes, sometimes bleeding and sneezing attacks, sometimes so bad that I couldn't sleep. When the problems got even worse after I bought a new laundry detergent, a light bulb went on. I thought then I was making a safe choice with the common perfume-free products found at the supermarket or drugstore, but this was not the case. So it wasn't just the perfume, but also the synthetic substances used in the product. I went looking on the Internet, trying to find out what else could be the cause, and I mostly found information on American websites. At the time there wasn't a single Dutch-language website about MCS, which was especially bad considering that MCS must be recognized as soon as possible, so people can take measures to prevent worse from happening. At the time, providing information about the condition MCS was my motivation for putting www.mcs-allergie.info online.

Adjusting your life to MCS isn't always easy, and when your family and friends think it's all in your head, it doesn't make it any less complicated. I realize very well that it's not easy for many people to imagine that chemical substances and scents can make you sick. By talking with people and looking for solutions, you can often come to terms. But some people are incorrigible, for when you come over, the electric perfume dispenser will still be running, or they'll come to your birthday dinner bringing flowers which I absolutely can't tolerate. In my experience, especially, family members have trouble taking your requests seriously, because after all, you didn't always have those problems!

MCS contributed to the decision to move, since having a dry cleaner in the neighborhood was too unhealthy. And now my problems have been reduced to an acceptable level. I can have people visit or go to a dance class a few times per week, but I can't work outside the home. With my kids growing up, I did want to start doing something again. Visitors to my website often asked me questions in the guest book about where in the Netherlands they could purchase safe products. Many safe products come from other countries, which isn't convenient for many people. I thus started an online store: the Sensitive Shop, www.sensitiveshop.nl. This has been going for some years now and I enjoy doing it. More and more people with sensitivities are finding the Sensitive Shop and often I get nice responses. In this way I try to find a healthy balance in my life with MCS, to adjust my life as much as possible and, above all, come to terms with having MCS. Aside from that, it's of course best to accept when some people don't want to believe you and to just focus on your own efforts to continue your own (adjusted) life as normally as possible.

121. Theo, 56

Over twelve years ago I became sick. Since I was twenty-five I worked in an operating room; the work consisted mostly of ear, nose, throat and jaw surgery. Many children came in for their tonsils and of course we used a lot of narcotic gas. After reorganization led to a transfer to a different operating room, I was sick for three quarters of a year and then stayed at home for half a year. The first diagnosis was hypothyroidism (the insufficient production of thyroid hormone by the thyroid gland). After using the medicine Thyrax my body recovered and I was able to return to work.

Measurements taken at my workplace indicated that the ventilation was barely functioning, allowing chemical substances and gases to accumulate too much. Within a year I was once again very sick with very diverse complaints: pain everywhere, heart palpitations, high blood pressure, intestinal problems, skin problems, difficulty thinking, and so on. Coincidentally my internal specialist read an article in the newspaper about chronic toxic encephalopathy (CTE or psycho-organic syndrome).

This is a disease caused by exposure to toxic solvents or substances such as paint. He said I might have this disease. Several visits then took place, to a neurologist, a psychologist, a neuro-psychologist and a homeopathic therapist, and the result was that it could be CTE due to toxic exposure to Halothane. This is a liquid gas used for anesthesia in the operating room. From this day on I've been working hard, trying to collect as much information and knowledge on the subject as possible. This persistence has come about because while I was sick, many made me out to be crazy. They said the similarity to CTE was incorrect. By now I know better.

After a long while I went back to my workplace, but within a day was back at square one. I later discovered this is a normal reaction.

In later phases of my illness I became sensitive to more substances: first paint, then amalgam, pesticides, herbicides and car exhaust. The last sensitivities to join the list were perfumes and other scent substances. You can try to avoid many things, but unfortunately these scents substances are found almost everywhere and there is barely any sympathy for this kind of problem.

Due to all these problems I can no longer practice my old trade and I eventually changed jobs, so I would no longer have to work with narcotic gases. But I still have to deal with my chemical sensitivity to various substances and scents every day.

Website: www.safer-world.org/nl/ Prive%20ervaringen/theo.htm

122. Anonymous, 75

Ever since childhood I've had various allergies and sensitivities, especially to food. I had rhinitis, skin problems and several other conditions. I am convinced the foundation for various sensitivities, just like MCS, is genetic. Certain enzymes are missing which normally ensure that toxic substances can be removed from the body. If you do not have these enzymes, or if they are damaged, then you'll be in trouble if you are exposed to too many chemicals in your life.

My parents ran a barbershop and from an early age onwards I would help out. It was assumed I would eventually take over. But when I started getting problems with the liquids for hair perms and, a number of years later, with the hair dyes, that was ruled out and eventually I totally stepped out of it. I developed eczema and welts on my skin from using those substances, and could only cut or comb people's hair. This of course was quite limited. I once had to undergo two operations in short order, and had to swallow a number of antibiotics courses in order to rid myself of an infection that followed. These antibiotics have permanently damaged my mucous membranes internally and externally. Because of my various allergies and strange reactions to substances I ended up at the hospital with an allergist, who wanted to do extensive testing on me. A few days later I fell into a coma just like that, probably as a result of an allergic reaction to the tests. The coma did not leave me entirely undamaged; after this incident I started reacting very sensitively to all kinds of synthetic substances, including perfume, deodorant, and laundry products. As soon as I am exposed to these substances, I get blisters in my mouth as well as skin problems, primarily itchiness and welts.

For this reason I now avoid chemical substances as much as possible. This makes it hard for me to have a normal social life, go visit people or entertain guests. I only see my son every once in a while and only outside, because he smokes and I can't handle the chemicals that he carries with him. I have my groceries delivered to me at home and I'm basically always at home and am usually lying on the bed because I have problems sitting (a painful bottom due to medications in the past). I really need household help, but I can't find anyone, because nobody is willing to come without wearing perfumes, so for better or worse I try to do things myself.

Because I have scoliosis, I walk with a limp. I need a hip operation, but can no longer tolerate medicine. Because of my sensitivity to many other chemical substances I would be hopping from the frying pan into the fire, so I won't have it done. My specialist also advised me not to do so with regard to my skin conditions.

Because of the health problems in my youth I do luckily have a relatively high tolerance for suffering, but things are getting harder as I get older, especially as an MCS patient, because I simply can't get help. Nothing has been arranged for MCS patients. I hope that one day there will be a special building or a special neighborhood with only MCS-safe apartments and houses, as well as health care adapted to MCS patients. But that's all in the future and it's likely to be quite some time before this happens. For now I must play the hand I was dealt. It is what it is.

In Memory of Deceased MCS Patients

123. Andrea Voerman, 1956–2004

Andrea suffered from various allergies during her entire life. As a baby she already had problems with breast milk, for example. Due to enzyme deficiencies she developed a muscle disorder. From the age of twenty onwards the condition left her more and more disabled, until she became dependent on a wheelchair at the age of twenty-nine. Allergies were common on both sides of her family and she herself was sensitive to many substances, especially foods (including all kinds of cereals). She had to feed herself liquid foods using a stomach tube and relied on a diet entirely adjusted to her allergies. She had to adhere to a strict rotary diet, so she could still eat certain vegetables, for example.

Eventually the chemical sensitivity surfaced just as all kinds of strongly perfumed laundry products hit the market. She started noticing that every time a strongly perfumed friend came to visit, it would make her sick. Over the years she became an ever more severe MCS patient who ended up in complete isolation. Even the chemical substances that later often were processed in sheets and clothing caused great problems, such as very serious ear infections. Her parents took loving care of her and made sure that she was exposed to

harmful substances as little as possible. Because of this they also lost a part of the family that could not sympathize with and understand the situation. When she was forty-two years old, her muscle disease left her bedridden and dependent on help. The Dutch home care system did not come through. There was ample budget, but little to no perfume-free help was offered, the reason being that it could not be "negotiated."

Due to complete exhaustion caused by the intense pain that she suffered (which also kept her from sleeping) and the many medications she had to take (which barely helped her at all), Andrea passed away at the age of forty-eight. Her body completely caved in, according to her parents. Her spirit as well seemed to have given up, after having displayed an enormous strength for years. Despite everything, she went forth peacefully, and for this her parents are grateful.

124. Cindy Deuhring, 1962–1999

Cindy was a student, athlete and musician, who hoped to one day become a doctor. But her plans fell to pieces when she became incurably ill after being exposed to a high dose of pesticides. She was in her last year of college when a cleaning service treated her apartment with pesticides in order to fight fleas. From that moment on Cindy struggled with her deteriorating health. She was eventually a prisoner in her own home, entirely sealed in with a constantly running air purifier. In the following years her life became very complicated as she kept on having to further isolate herself from the world. She reacted extremely sensitively to low doses of chemical substances. Even the most modern appliances such as a telephone, a radio or a computer were eventually no longer possible for her to use. Everything made her sick. In time, her organs could no longer take it and, as a result of MCS, she passed away at a very early age. www.ciin.org/pages/04-fund.html

125. Julia Kendall 1935–1997

Julia became sick from the pesticide malathion, as a result of which she had to adapt her life. She became an activist in the field of the poisonous effects of chemicals on the health of humans, and an experienced anti-pesticide advocate. In 1994 she led the campaign against an American airline, urging it to stop the unreported misting of passengers with pesticides. This generated a lot of publicity and led to the end of these kinds of practices in various countries. She organized many demonstrations and campaigns as well as publicizing lawsuits against the manufacturers of poisonous products. She strongly believed that these industries are not as powerful as they seem. If consumers stop buying

their products or if their shares are no longer traded, they will be forced to either improve or go out of business. She was an unstoppable researcher of people who had been injured by chemicals and shared her fountain of knowledge and enormous database with everyone who might need it. Julia Kendall died from complications arising from leukemia. www.ourlittleplace.com/julia. html; http://users.lmi.net/~wilworks/ newreact/julia97.htm

126. Domenic Troiano, 1932–1999

Domenic and his wife both fell seriously ill after they moved into a recently remodeled home. (See *entry 96* for their story.) Before Domenic got sick, he played in a band. He was a great singer and loved to dance. Peggy and Domenic used to dance three or four times each week. They liked to travel and spent many days on the water, as Domenic had his captain's license and was also a fisherman. Out of their love for water, they chose the name "MCS, beacon of hope" for the foundation. Peggy and Domenic had promised one another that if one would survive MCS longer than the other, the survivor would do everything they could to help others in the same boat, or to prevent chemicals from injuring more people. Thus "MCS" Beacon of Hope was created. Domenic died as a result of his advanced MCS on 3 January 1999. http://mcsbeac onofhope.com/in_loving_memory. htm

127. Dan Allen, 1956–2004

Dan Allen, a football coach, developed MCS as a result of renovations made to the field house on the campus of Holy Cross College. A new floor had been laid, and the gases, the chemicals and the other harmful substances in the air that entered his office made him ill. He started experiencing various symptoms and began reacting to chemical substances. His neuromuscular system was weakened with every exposure to hazardous substances. Instead of running across the sports fields, he could no longer do so and increasingly had to use a golf cart or a cane. Allen ended up in a wheelchair. In 2003 he was replaced with a different coach. Dan Allen's injuries included toxic encephalopathy, respiratory problems and a lung condition, symptoms of poisoning, and chronic fatigue.

Although Dan had been diagnosed with MCS, this was not reported in his official death certificate. His death is officially the result of a "neuromuscular degeneration" (a disease that damages the nervous system and muscles). No autopsy was performed. www.ridefor life.com/news/als_news/multiple_ chemical_sensitivity_and_als.html

128. Kim Palmer, 1954–2006

Kim Palmer was a singer and songwriter in the United States who developed MCS after experiencing a small gas leak in her apartment, which was not discovered until two years later. In those two years her health significantly deteriorated. She slept with the windows shut in a room that had just been painted, she worked with pesticides, and she had torn up a very moldy carpet after a flood, all of which in combination with the gas leak conspired to make her a severe MCS patient. After years of searching for an MCS-safe place to live, she wound up in an RV in the Arizona desert, where she kept writing her songs. Her CD *Songs from a Porcelain Trailer* is an MCS product inspired by this experience. See *entry 334*.

In the end her body succumbed to the many health problems she had developed. Kim passed away at a young age. www.kimpalmersongs.com; www.angel fire.com/az/ox/kim-palmer-story.html; http://home.datacomm.ch/rezamusic/ tv.html

129. Elizabeth Hope Streightif, 1945–2004

In 1983 Elizabeth was exposed to chemical solvents, which made her very sensitive to very many chemicals, pesticides, and solvents. For the twenty years that followed she was in a constant battle against MCS, always looking for a safe house and for the right treatment that could make her better. The last two years of her life were the hardest. She became weaker and weaker and the doctors just couldn't discover what was causing it. Eventually they found a perforated colon and she underwent an operation, which was followed by a period of chronic infections. She lost all her strength and could no longer walk or sit up for long. She passed through various hospitals. Eventually, a stroke brought an end to her life. http://immuneweb. org/immunites/bets.html

130. Nancy Noren, 1947–1998

Nancy was a normal, healthy and athletic woman who worked as a systems analyst before she developed MCS. For the first five years of her illness, she was confined to her house and totally incapable of functioning. She eventually moved to New Mexico where the air was cleaner and where other MCS patients had gone as well. There she was able to function again, as long as she did not get exposed to pesticides, which would totally disable her. Unfortunately, her neighbors refused to warn her when they planned to spray pesticides. She wasn't able to close her windows in time, and suffered immensely due to the inflexible attitude of these neighbors. On bad days, when there were pesticide fumes, she would flee her house and head into nature in a trailer. But she could usually not stay in campsites, due to the chemical substances found there (such as charcoal lighter fluid and cleaning products in the bathrooms), so she often camped out in the wilderness on a remote mesa. It was on such a mesa

that Nancy was killed by a 22-year-old man, who was later arrested in her truck. His notes revealed that he had been stalking her in the wilderness for some time. www.accessmylibrary.com/ coms2/summary_0286-431787_ITM

131. Irene Ruth Wilkenfeld, 1945–2004

Irene Wilkenfeld became ill when she was exposed to Chlordane (a pesticide) at the school at which she taught. In 1987 her MCS worsened after she moved into a newly constructed building. The formaldehyde and the other toxic substances that the new materials gassed out made her very sick. For the rest of her life Irene worked to inform others and teach about the dangers of pesticides. She also educated many people and made them aware of how important it is that children have a safe, healthy environment at school. Irene Wilkenfeld died as a result of liver failure. Her work has helped many people, and she left a powerful statement in her will, which you can read online. www.head-gear.com/SafeSchools/eth will.html; www.mcscanadian.org/mem oriam.html; www.head-gear.com/Safe Schools/irene.html

13

Links to Websites with More Testimonies

132. The Wall of Personal Testimony

www.herc.org/wall

133. Chemical Illness Report Page

www.chem-tox.com/guest-whistle/guestbook.html

134. MCS-international: Meet the Team

www.mcs-international.org/about_us/meet_the_team.html

135. Gathering Stories about Chemical Injury

www.citlink.net/~bhima/gathering.htm

136. "No Safe Haven: People with MCS Are Becoming the New Homeless"

www.emagazine.com/view/?1003

137. Read These People's Stories, Then Consider This ... Could You Be Next?

www.mcs-global.org/Stories.htm

138. Personal Stories from MCS Patients around the EHC-Dallas

www.ehcd.com/websteen/ehcd_patient_stories.htm

139. Share a Day in Your Life with Chronic Illness

http://planetthrive.com/cgi-bin/members/pub9990215236064.cgi

140. Aroma of Christ: Faces of the Chemically Sensitive

www.aromaofchrist.com/Faces%20of%20MCS%20Title%20Page.htm

PART IV

The ABCs of MCS: Tips and Advice in Alphabetical Order

A number of points of interest with regard to this chapter:

• In cases where the author discusses specific physical symptoms of MCS and possible treatments for them, it is assumed that the reader has already sought and/or received regular medical attention and that the ailments/symptoms are clearly a result of MCS and are not based in any other medical condition.

• The author is not responsible for the consequences of carrying out informal tips, which are usually informed by her own experiences. See the Disclaimer in the beginning of this book.

• No MCS patient is the same; this means that the products mentioned in this book are not necessarily suitable for everyone. It's a matter of finding out what works for you. Always be careful when trying tips and advice from others;

indeed, this applies to all tips and advice in this book as well. The author merely hopes to extend a helping hand to MCS patients in need.

• No commercial interest is involved in the mention of certain companies and/or retail outlets. Such references are merely intended as information; as of this writing, there are very few retail outlets for MCS products.

• Although the author strived to be as complete as possible when compiling this section, undoubtedly certain items and issues were overlooked. Experiences, tips, and so on can be passed on to the author (valkenburg@the-abc-of-mcs.nl) and may be included in possible new editions of this book and/or posted on the website www.the-abc-of-mcs.com.

141. Activated charcoal

Activated charcoal, also known as activated carbon, is used to remove various chemical substances from the air. It is used, among other things, in masks, rugs (in a closet, for example) and in air purifiers. Conventional air purifiers often use activated carbon, but usually this is insufficient for an MCS patient. Impregnated carbon generally works much better, because it can bind itself to more substances and therefore cleans more substances from the air. (*Impregnated* implies that a porous solid substance is drenched in a liquid to protect the product and, in this case, to improve its efficiency.) For this reason most air purifiers suitable for MCS use impregnated carbon rather than activated carbon.

For more information on the differences between the charcoals, see: http://science.howstuffworks.com/question209.htm.

Also see *entry 144.*

142. Air fresheners

Chemical air fresheners are certainly a large burden on an MCS patient, but even for healthy people these kinds of products are not recommended. Various studies have explored the consequences of using air fresheners, yielding controversial yet contradictory results. You can retrieve plenty of information on the subject through Google.

Every household can easily do without these artificial scent products. If you really need something to clear the air, you might think about ventilation (during hours when the outside air is clean enough), an air purifier, or — for small, enclosed spaces — putting some baking soda in a bowl to absorb the smells. Dried herbs, flowers or essential oils can also help.

See the article "Air Fresheners (or 'Air Poisoners'?)" at www.ourlittleplace.com/air.html.

143. Air pollution

On the website www.the-abc-of-mcs.com and in *Part VI* of this book you can find maps of the worst-polluted places in the world. These maps can help if you're making plans to move. Yet these maps often only indicate part of the existing pollution, and other areas might have different problems —fires and stoves, for example, are lit just about everywhere. If you're planning on moving, solid preparation and thorough research are a necessity to avoid jumping from the frying pan into the fire!

144. Air purifiers

There are various MCS-appropriate air purifiers. These are geared towards MCS patients as much as possible. Yet of course it's always a matter of testing to see if a particular purifier is right for you. You can often take a purifier home for testing before buying it. Do keep in mind that no matter which air purifier you use, you should first let it run in another room in order to blow out all the "start-up gases."

Below you will find a summation of the air purifying systems which currently tend to work best for MCS patients. You can also get information from other MCS patients by joining an online MCS group.

1. *AllerAir AirMedic MCS Series Air Purifiers* (www.achooallergy.com/allera ir-airmedic-mcs-mscd-airpurifiers.asp) *Austin Air Healthmate + (Superblend) Air Purifier* (www.achooallergy.com/ austinhealthmate-superblend.asp). These two devices are specifically made for MCS patients, especially in terms of the filter materials used, the steel housing, the use of an unbleached, pesticide-free cotton pre-filter and granular activated charcoal. This filter device can purify more gases from the air than active carbon can. You can request the filter specifications from a supplier. Several suppliers sell these devices. The links contain much information and details about several air purifiers.

2. IQAir Multigas GC (www.iqair. com/EU/ENG/Products/GCSeries. htm). This is probably the best machine for MCS patients (after it has been properly out-gassed). This device is specifically designed for MCS patients. It uses relatively safe materials such as organic glue. This doesn't mean, though, that it is immediately suitable for everyone. According to the experiences of MCS patients, it's best to let a new device run for a long time (a few weeks or more, depending on your own sensitivity) in a room you do not have to enter and where the windows can be opened, until the gases from the new motor are gone. Your patience will be rewarded with an excellent machine once it is safe for you to use. Using a combination of the filter media VOC and Chemisorber (hence the name "Multigas") the device is able to purify an in-

credible amount of chemical substances. The filter medium consists of granular active carbon and aluminum oxide, impregnated with potassium permanganate (KMnO4). You can also order separate filter packs with granulate that can purify things like ammonia (useful in case you live in a rural area, with regard to manure). You can request the filter specifications from your supplier. Exchanging the filters is quite a quick and simple process and so you can even make combinations of the four filter packs yourself.

The IQair has various accessories, such as the Inflow W125. This item can slightly pressurize any given room, sucking air from outside through an aluminum hose and purifying it. This requires a hole to be made in the wall for the air supply component to which the IQair and the hose are then connected. For more information go to: www.achoo allergy.com/airpurifierattachments.asp, www.achooallergy.com/iqairpurifiers.asp and www.achooallergy.com/IQAIRGC GCX.asp.

3. *Amaircare Roomaid* (www.allergy asthmatech.com/P/Amaircare_Roomaid /593_315) (www.achooallergy.com/ro omaid.asp). This is a small air purifier which can be connected to the cigarette lighter in a car. It's hardy when traveling or in small rooms. The device can also be connected to the electric grid using a special plug and cable, which can be additionally ordered. It's advisable to also order the VOC canister, which purifies the air of smog, smoke, exhaust and other fumes. This purifier likely needs some time to gas out before using.

Additional information on other systems:

Air purifiers using only a HEPA filter:

These do not work for MCS patients, or at least not well, because they purify hardly any harmful chemical substances from the air. HEPA filters are mostly used to clean allergens, pollen, dust and spores of mold from the air.

Air purifiers using only active carbon:

These do purify chemical substances from the air, but active carbon alone usually doesn't satisfy the needs of an MCS patient. Impregnated carbon (whereby a chemical particle has been added to the carbon) augments the purifying capacity. For this reason almost all MCS air purifiers use a filter medium made of impregnated carbon.

Ionizers:

Ionizers, which purify the air using negative ions, are usually not tolerated well by MCS patients because they create ozone. Small ionizers are sometimes good to use for de-scenting a drawer, closet, car, or any other small space, but they do still release a small amount of ozone into the air. You can read more information about ionizers at http://en.wikipedia.org/wiki/Air_ioniser.

Portable ionizer:

Sometimes small ionizers are worn around the neck — for example, during traveling — because these are supposed to neutralize smoke, pollen and certain gases. Often an ionizer is used with a cotton MCS mask. Do not keep the device close enough to smell the ozone, because it can be very irritating to your nostrils or cause a reaction. The ionizer will help only when you sit still in an area with air that is not moving. Make sure you can tolerate this before you use it. For more information, see www.negativeiongenerators.com/portableairpurifier.html and www.natlallergy.com/product.asp?pn=1121&bhcd2=12251043 78.

Powered Air Purifying Respirator (PAPR):
See *entry 274.*

145. Alcohol

ALCOHOLIC BEVERAGES

Consuming alcoholic beverages is not advisable for MCS patients. Many MCS patients have an impaired detoxification system, which means alcohol is just another burden upon the liver. Some patients immediately have a reaction when they drink alcohol, and others notice that even just one drink leaves them with an extreme hangover, because their body does not respond well.

When breaking down alcohol, your liver produces the poisonous substance acetaldehyde. Because the body of an MCS patient already has trouble tolerating and processing harmful substances, it's not a good idea to consume alcohol.

ISOPROPYL ALCOHOL

According to a tip posted to a Canadian forum, isopropyl alcohol (99 percent) can apparently remove perfume scents from clothing, sheets, and so on. According to this tip, you should soak the clothing in a large bucket of water, along with ¼ to ½ cup of alcohol (make a weak solution). Then rinse the clothing and wash it as you normally would, a number of times if necessary. Just to be safe, you could also hang up the clothes for a few days so they can air out before you use them. During this whole process, protect yourself against the vapors with gloves and a respirator, because isopropyl alcohol is toxic. This kind of alcohol is not for internal use! Labeled as rubbing alcohol, 99 percent isopropyl alcohol is sold in pharmacies.

146. Allerair Air Purifier

See *entry 144.*

147. Allergies

Aside from the fact that chemical substances make them sick, some MCS patients also develop allergies and food intolerances. It's best to let yourself be treated by a therapist or doctor who can test for such things. Here, too, avoidance is the best "medicine," as opposed to using all sorts of medications intended to suppress the allergic reactions (although in cases of anaphylactic shock, medicine is a matter of life and death!). Allergy and food intolerance treatment now includes a number of methods, such as low-dose antigen therapy (LDA), enzyme-potentiated desensitization (EPD neutralization injections) and the provocation/neutralization method (injections).

Not every allergic MCS patient responds well to these lengthy treatments. They are intensive and usually do not resolve MCS problems, but they do work to reduce allergic reactions (IgE). These can be very expensive, so make sure you are well informed before undergoing treatments in this field. To read more about allergies and chemical reactions, see http://mcs-america.org/ziemallergiesmcs.pdf. For more information on EPD and LDA, go to www.dma.org/~rohrers/allergy/epd_faq.htm and www.drshrader.com/pr02.htm.

148. Aluminum foil

In general aluminum foil is easily tolerated by MCS patients and can be used for all sorts of purposes, even things like covering an unsafe wall or wrapping particle board. Aluminum foil could also be used for protection from electro smog, and it's better than plastic for wrapping food.

149. Aluminum foil tape

Aluminum foil tape is primarily used to seal off openings and to cover plastics or other synthetic substances so as to prevent them from releasing gases. Aluminum tape is available from Amazon.com and many other businesses (search "aluminum foil tape" on Google). Make sure you protect yourself when using this tape, because its glue may cause a reaction.

150. Amaircare Roomaid

See *entry 144.*

151. Amalgam

Many MCS patients have the amalgam removed from their teeth in the hope that this will relieve their MCS. It is often asserted in various alternative health communities that the safe removal of amalgam has a positive effect on one's general well-being. Some people notice a big difference after taking this step; others notice nothing at all. For MCS patients, as far as we know, removing all amalgam fillings is not a solution or a cure for their chemical sensitivity problems. For the general burden on the body, however, it can be better to have the amalgam removed, since the mercury that is released when teeth come together or when the amalgam wears down can be taxing on the body. The process of amalgam removal is not entirely without risk for an MCS patient, so it should be done with utmost care. It should be carried out in small steps and with very solid protection, such as a dental dam. (See http://en.wikipedia.org/wiki/Dental_dam for more information.) One should, of course, also consider alternatives, such as porcelain, gold, or composite. Treatments from a dentist can in general make an MCS patient temporarily sicker; using tri-salts is also advisable. See *entry 302* for information about tri-salts. Also see *entry 180* about visits to the dentist and options for anesthesia.

For more information on the materials used and specific dental/dentist information for MCS patients go to: http://stason.org/TULARC/health/dental-amalgam/13-Is-There-Information-For-Chemically-Sensitive-Patient.html.

152. Anaphylactic shock

Anaphylactic shock is a *severe allergic reaction with the risk of a fatal outcome* if there is not a timely response. Anaphylactic shock is characterized by severe shortness of breath due to (among other things): constriction of the airways, accumulation of moisture under the skin, and sudden severe loss of blood pressure. In order to neutralize the reaction, an injection of adrenaline is necessary, for example using an EpiPen.

If there is any inkling of anaphylactic shock, *immediately call 911: medical help is absolutely necessary and can be lifesaving!!!* The best thing is to administer rescue breathing until the ambulance or medical aid arrives. Find more information about anaphylaxis at www.foodallergy.org.

153. Austin Air

See *entry 144.*

154. Baking soda

Baking soda is a white powder, properly called sodium bicarbonate, which can be used both internally and externally. (*Baking soda is not the same as Borax; Borax, also known as sodium borate, is very poisonous when consumed!*) Baking soda can be used in foods in very small amounts, for example as a raising agent. When dissolved in a glass of water, it is sometimes used as an antacid. Always first read the instructions for use on the packaging in order to use the right amount.

In larger amounts baking soda can be used for other purposes, for example as a disinfecting and cleaning agent, as softener, or for small infected cuts, for example. MCS patients have flocked to baking soda because it's a good deodorizer (add it to the washing machine or place it in a bowl in a small room). Some MCS patients also use it as a laundry detergent. You can add small amounts of baking soda to your bath (for detoxification or treating itchiness), use it as a deodorant (powder it on as you would talcum powder) and even for extra dental care (dissolve one teaspoon in a glass of water and rinse forcefully). Baking soda binds acids and lowers the acid content of the body, which raises the pH value. A higher pH value (alkaline base instead of acidic) allows chemical substances to be processed and carried off more easily. In case of liver or coronary problems, or high blood pressure, baking soda treatment should *always* be discussed with your doctor before use. Do not use too much, especially internally. For regular internal use to neutralize reactions to chemicals or alkalize, tri-salts are preferable because tri-salts do not contain sodium. (Also see *entry 302* and www.needs.com/product/Ecological_Formulas_Tri_Salts_200/b_Ecological_Formulas.)

Baking soda can be purchased at health food stores, supermarkets (located among the baking products, like flour or baking powder), drug stores or a pharmacies.

155. Barbecues

Barbecuing is often no longer possible for MCS patients, who may get sick from the fumes that are released. You can still use an electric grill, but make sure that you're sitting upwind as these too will release fumes. Also see *entry 291.*

156. Bedding

You should always tackle your bedroom first, making it completely chemical-free and only using properly gassed-out and all-organic materials, especially the mattress. Several stores sell organic bedding and other items; see *Part VI* for addresses or visit the website www.the-abc-of-mcs.com.

157. Bionase Nasal Applicator

Bionase is a device specifically designed for patients with hay fever that reduces the sensitivity and hyperreactivity of the nasal mucous membrane. Bionase works using light therapy, which makes the mucous membrane in the nose less irritable. This can weaken one's sensitivity, especially to allergies. For MCS patients it can be beneficial by making the nasal mucous membrane smaller and thus creating more space for the air supply. This can prevent infections and clogged noses. Harmful substances should certainly still be avoided. For further information, see www.intelligenthealthsystems.com.au/bionase.htm and www.smartmiracles.com/p-Gifts-75-100/BS511/Bionase+Nasal+Applicator.html.

158. Biotensor

A biotensor is an instrument that is used much like a pendulum to test the energy flow in the body. Yet a biotensor does not look like a pendulum: it has a handle and a long antenna with at the end either a ball, a spiral or a circle. The biotensor is used by various natural healers and alternative therapists for all kinds of testing and research, for example in cases of food allergies and/or food combinations, vitamins, minerals, homeopathy, and diet advice, among others. The person holding the instrument is actually doing the measuring and sensing; the biotensor is merely the translator. The biotensor or pendulum thus works as an antenna that picks up signals. Some consider it an extension of the subconscious.

If you'd like to start using a biotensor yourself, it's recommended that you first study up on how it works, because you run the risk of divining falsehoods. This has to do with the fact that what lives inside of you is crystallized through the biotensor, which makes it possible that the biotensor is actually relaying your own fears and convictions. Also see http://pendulumsplus.com/biotensor-professional br32-p-60.html.

159. Blood pressure

Low blood pressure can make you lethargic, tired, foggy in the head and dizzy. If you are dealing with low blood pressure, drinking licorice root tea (if this can be tolerated) is a good and healthy alternative way to tackle the problem.

Excessive use, however, risks the flip side of the problem, namely that your blood pressure can run high. It can also cause other side effects. See www.herbsarespecial.com.au/free-herb-information/licorice.html for more information.

If you experience side effects with one cup a day, you are clearly intolerant to it and you should immediately stop drinking this tea.

It's best to have your blood pressure checked regularly, or you can buy a reliable meter for home use. In case of high blood pressure, consult your general practitioner. Often it's a matter of adjusting your diet and lifestyle, and in some cases medication is necessary.

160. Books

See *entry 221.*

161. Borax

Borax is also known as sodium borate, *but is not the same as baking soda: borax is very poisonous, especially when consumed!!!* Borax is nonetheless sometimes used by MCS patients as an alternative for cleaning or dish detergents, or as a disinfecting or bleaching substance. It is also used as a laundry detergent or fabric softener. Borax is a powerful substance and, when mixed with lemon juice into a paste, is an excellent cleaning substance for the toilet bowl: apply paste, let it soak for two hours, and scrub with a brush. Watch out for splashing!

Borax must not be taken internally. Borax is very toxic to the nervous system, the kidneys and the liver. It can be absorbed through damaged skin, and when it comes in contact with skin it can cause sensitive reactions. Inhaling the powder can also irritate the airways, among other things. If you want to use borax, always protect yourself. To dissolve it, stir the borax into warm water. Remember that borax is primarily used as a strong disinfectant or to kill all sorts of vermin in the home and garden. Most grocery stores sell Borax in the cleaning section or the laundry aisle. More details and information on Borax can be found at www.safe2use.com/scabiesboard/borax.htm.

162. Brain fog

"Brain fog" is a term used to describe the feeling of having clouds in your head — as if wads of cotton are in your head. Brain fog usually arises after exposure to an irritant and primarily causes concentration problems. By consistently avoiding the instigating substances, brain fog can be mitigated. You can play some funny mind-stimulating games at www.naturescountrystore.com/canaryrehab/index.html.

163. Business cards

In order to provide others with information on MCS, it's useful to refer them to the website www.the-abc-of-mcs.com. On this site you'll find various articles, links and information on MCS. On this site you'll also find (under the heading "Miscellaneous") business cards which you are free to use. It's best to have someone else print these cards on thick paper; when the printouts have been gassed out, the cards can be cut to size. Especially if you walk outside wearing a mask or a helmet, it's very useful to be able to hand out an informational card when you are asked questions. This will keep you from having to explain yourself repeatedly, and you'll be able to go on with what you were doing.

164. Cables and fittings

New cables and recently coated fittings can cause problems. Always keep some old or gassed-out cables, fittings and wires in your shed or storage area; often it can take months before a new cable is properly gassed out. An alternative is to wrap the cable with aluminum foil tape; see *entry 149*.

165. Caffeine

Most MCS patients do not respond well to caffeine. A good alternative is to choose an organic coffee purchased in a natural foods store that has been made caffeine-free by a process using water (see, for example, www.coffeelover susa.com/organic-decaf.html). Most decaf coffee is decaffeinated using chemicals, so "regular" decaf is certainly not recommended for an MCS patient.

166. Candida

Candida is a genus of yeast that when allowed to grow excessively, can lead to a (vaginal) yeast infection. This yeast infection can arise in MCS patients from time to time. Anal itching is also often a sign that there is too much *Candida* in the intestines.

When possible, it is best to prevent or treat it with natural remedies, such as organic tea tree oil (use only externally) and Molkosan (rinse vaginally after diluting it on a ratio of 1:4). These treatments are effective ways to suppress a beginning infection, but if the infection is advanced, a medicinal ointment can be necessary (ask your general practitioner for advice). In case of a persistent or repeated yeast infections, it's advisable to get in touch with an experienced therapist.

In order to prevent a yeast infection, it's recommended that, among other things, you eat as little sugar as possible and maintain an anti–*Candida* diet. Various resources on the subject can be found online. See: www.medicinenet. com/yeast_vaginitis/article.htm, www. thecandidadiet.com.

Here are links to some products which, when tolerated, can be helpful:

Gy-na-Tren (oral and vaginal capsules): http://natrenpro.com/product_gy-na-tren.asp

Molkosan: www.herbsmd.com/deta il/Molkosan-20811.htm

Organic Tea Tree Oil: www.911health shop.com/orteatreoilb.html

Reusable vaginal douche: www.amaz on.com/Cara-Douche-Syringe-Bulb-Lu xury/dp/B0012JZVIO

Threelac: www.candidayeastinfecti on.com

167. Candles

The smoke from candles can cause problems even if they're not scented or colored candles. If you'd still like an element of coziness in your home, it's a good idea to make the switch to the very pleasant electronic candles, such as those sold by: www.norexbuydir ect.com.

168. Car travel

First of all, it's not advisable for an MCS patient to make use of a new car, because the profusion of synthetic materials emits many gases. In particular, the softening agents (phthalates) in the synthetic materials can cause problems. Don't get this one wrong!

When shopping for a car, it's best to choose among secondhand cars in which the former owners neither smoked nor sprayed perfume. When buying a used car, be sure to make it clear to the dealership that they mustn't use chemical substances to fix the car up and give it that "wonderful just-like-new smell"! If you already own a car, it's good to have a HEPA (white) and an active carbon (black) filter installed so that all the air blown into the car through the air conditioning system will first pass through these filters. The active carbon removes exhaust fumes from the air while the HEPA filter stops soot particles, pollen, and so forth. During your car's annual checkup you will then have these filters replaced. If your car does not have an inbuilt option to install filters, a car mechanic can often put something together and order and install the filters separately. Ask your auto repair center for advice and solutions. If no filter is suitable for your car, you can always use the portable air purifier inside the car (see next paragraph).

In traffic jams and on busy roads, push the "recycle" button so that air will temporarily circulate within the car instead of polluted air being supplied from outside. There is also a special air purifier for use inside the car (see *entry 144*) which is powered by the cigarette lighter outlet. You can also order an additional box of active carbon in order to increase the capacity of the HEPA air purifier.

You can use the motor of the Powered Air Purifying Respirator (PAPR) (see *entry 274*), keeping it on your lap to ensure a constant supply of purified air. In general, maintain a lot of distance between you and the cars in front of you and avoid rush hour traffic. Definitely have someone else fill your car with gas or wear a mask while filling up (or drive an electric car).

169. Cardiac arrhythmia

Cardiac arrhythmia can arise due to exposure to chemicals, but also due to certain deficiencies in the body. A magnesium deficiency, for example (common among MCS patients), can lead to heart palpitations and arrhythmia. Cardiac arrhythmia can also arise as a reaction to a food item or additive to which you have become sensitive or as a result of high blood pressure. A clinical specialist or therapist can test you for deficiencies.

170. Caulk

The safest caulks for MCS patients seem to be aquarium-safe caulk and Safecoat Caulk from AFM, because these types of caulk doesn't contain many of the additives other caulks do. Aquarium-safe caulk is used to glue aquariums and therefore does not contain solvents or other toxic substances. It is made of silicone, but when you have to do some caulking, it's probably the

best option. Here, too, you have to take the time to allow the caulk to gas out. Make sure you don't enter the space in which the caulk was used for a number of days. Aquarium caulks can be purchased in pet stores or in shops that sell aquariums, such as one: www.bigalsonline.com. You can also find it at some hardware stores. Look for a label that says "aquarium safe" or "safe for use on aquariums (100% clear silicone)."

For more on Safecoat Caulking Compound, see www.natureneutral.com.

171. Ceramic oxygen mask

It's recommended to purchase this mask if you have to use oxygen or if you don't want to use a plastic mask. This mask and the accompanying Tygon tubing can be purchased at www.aehf.com.

172. Chronic fatigue

MCS is characterized by different phases and many different symptoms. Chronic fatigue is a symptom of MCS. It's also common for patients with fibromyalgia and CFS to be chemically sensitive. Chronic exhaustion along with MCS can have many causes: small infections in the body, a yeast infection, sensitivity to electro smog, vitamin or mineral deficiency and, of course, chemical sensitivity. If the consistent avoidance of chemical substances does not bring about improvement, it's advisable to start researching other possible causes and to have yourself tested for a possible imbalance in vitamins, minerals and amino acids.

It's important to realize that chronic fatigue and chronic fatigue syndrome (CFS) are two entirely different issues: chronic fatigue is a symptom that arises with many illnesses; chronic fatigue syndrome (CFS) is a disease which includes not only fatigue but also other symptoms. One of the biggest misunderstandings is that people with CFS are simply tired. Another misunderstanding is that people who are tired have CFS. It's possible, of course, to have both MCS and CFS (they are considered partially overlapping conditions), but each must be diagnosed separately. Thus you can't conclude that someone who has MCS and is fatigued also has CFS.

Read more about CFS, MCS and overlapping diseases: www.satori-5.co. uk/word_articles/mcs/engaging_with_mcs.html. The U.S. Centers for Disease Control and Prevention provides information on CFS online at www.cdc.gov/cfs/pdf/Diagnosing_CFS.pdf and www. cdc.gov/cfs/cfssymptomsHCP.htm.

173. Cigarette smoke

As an MCS patient, make sure you never inhale cigarette smoke (including second-hand smoke). Cigarette smoke contains some four thousand chemicals that your body would then attempt to process. Cigarette smoke can be so irritating to your mucous membranes and lungs as to leave you with small infections. Every exposure can lead to a deterioration of your condition and increase the number of substances to which you react sensitively.

174. Cleaning products

It's often a challenge to find the right cleaning product or brand. MCS patients all react differently to the various options. It's just a matter of trying things out. For example, there are many MCS patients who are able to tolerate the brands Ecover or Seventh Generation well, while other MCS patients can't at all. It should go without saying that synthetic and perfumed cleaning products from the supermarket should be avoided as much as possible. Something that's a great tip for one person may be a disaster for someone else, so be careful when trying things out!

TIPS

• Vinegar offers many possibilities for use and can be purchased in natural foods stores and grocery stores. It's also good for wiping windows.
• A warm solution of baking soda and water is suitable for many cleaning needs and can be combined with white natural vinegar, for a good disinfecting agent.
• The combination of borax with lemon is also a good, strong alternative. A paste of lemon juice and borax is an excellent substance with which to clean the toilet bowl (apply pulp, let it soak for two hours, and scrub with toilet brush). Borax is also a good product for bleaching and disinfecting. Do not, however, confuse borax with baking soda! *When consumed or inhaled, borax is very toxic.* (Also see *entry 161*).
• Olive oil or almond oil is very suited to polishing wood furniture. There are also natural furniture polishes,

for example those sold through www.all naturalpolish.com.

Here are four very informative web-sites with alternative cleaning recipes. (Note: These are not specifically for MCS patients!):

www.ecologycenter.org/factsheets/cleaning.html
www.lesstoxicguide.ca/index.asp?fetch=household
http://recyclingnearyou.com.au/documents/2005125_natclean_eng.pdf
www.eartheasy.com/live_nontoxic_solutions.htm

175. Clothing

It's important to gas out new clothing and to wash new items a number of times before wearing them. Most cloth-ing is treated with many chemicals, such as pesticides on the cotton, bleach, syn-thetic paint, treatments in the produc-tion process and in the transportation containers, and so on. You should definitely not wear clothing that has just come from the dry cleaner, unless the dry cleaner does not use harmful chem-icals, in which case the clothes are prob-ably safe for MCS patients sooner. Be careful and well informed if you want to use this "green" alternative. "Green" does not necessarily mean it is also tol-erable or safe for MCS patients. See *Part VI* for web addresses on this subject.

Your best choice is to wear natural and organically produced cotton cloth-ing. For sources of clothing that is safer for MCS patients, visit www.the-abc-of-mcs.com.

176. Concentration, lack of

See *entry 162.*

177. Construction materials

Most new construction materials are not safe for use by MCS patients be-cause they contain chemical substances and release gases. Before you start build-ing or renovating, research your options and seek advice from experts in the field. In some situations it may be best to choose recycled construction materials; after all, these materials have usually al-ready gassed out. For more information on recycling, see www.neo.ne.gov/home_const/factsheets/recycled_const_mat.htm.

On The ABC of MCS website you can find various links which offer infor-mation on construction materials espe-cially suitable for MCS patients under the heading "Living."

In Dr. Rea's book (see *entry 328*) you can also find a list of construction ma-terials judged safe for MCS patients. The safest materials for MCS patients are, among others: glass, stone, steel, ce-ramic, aluminum, untreated hardwood and untreated natural products. How-ever, many kinds of wood can cause problems, particularly if the wood has been treated or impregnated, and some patients get sick from the resin which the wood may contain even when un-treated. White poplar wood is very suit-able for MCS patients, and is used, for example, in MCS saunas.

178. Cotton

Because cotton is extensively treated with chemicals during its growth/flowering, processing and transportation, it's best to opt for organic cotton whenever possible. Visit www.the-abc-of-mcs.com under the heading "Organic" for several addresses, or see *Part VI*.

179. Creativity

Aside from being a nice way to pass the time, keeping yourself busy in a creative or artistic way is a wonderful release for the various emotions which you will face as an MCS patient. If you plan on working with paint, however, you should make sure to take protective measures or to use as harmless a product as you can find.

Creativity can be expressed in many forms, including literature, art and music. Let your fellow "canaries" inspire you, for example in *Part V: Films, Books and Other Resources* of this book and through the international network for artists with MCS: www.creativecanaries.org. Through this network you can find a great deal of information on the use of safer materials.

180. Dentist

If you have a dental appointment, it's good to talk with your dentist about finding the safest way for you to visit. For example, you might ask beforehand that your dentist and his assistant refrain from wearing perfume or aftershave, and you can set a time for your visit so that you won't have to share the waiting room with other patients. If necessary, ask your dentist about the various options for anesthesia. Most MCS patients opt not to get amalgam placed in their teeth. Existing amalgam can be removed and replaced with porcelain, gold or composite fillings. See also *entry 151*.

Be aware that every treatment from a dentist will involve chemical substances. If you have negative side effects from the treatment, take tri-salts to neutralize the reaction (see *entry 302*). Consider seeing a holistic dentist, as this may increase your chances of finding a practice without perfume and the like. See the dentist referral list of MCS America: http://mcs-america.org/dentistlist.pdf. Be aware that not all the dentists on this list are familiar with MCS. Make sure you first talk with your potential new dentist about MCS and to see if he or she understands and respects your situation and can further help you.

Here is an informative link about going to a dentist as an MCS patient: http://stason.org/TULARC/health/dental-amalgam/13-Is-There-Information-For-The-Chemically-Sensitive-Patient.html.

181. Depression

Feelings of depression can be a result of exposure to chemical substances, so don't just think that everything is apparently too much for you to handle. Try avoiding chemical substances as much as possible and see what effect it has on your joy of life! It's also good to have your blood tested to see if any deficiencies have arisen, in magnesium for example (because this can definitely have an influence on your disposition). If the depression is persistent, seek guidance from an expert. A psychologist or a good therapist can help you get your life back on track despite your MCS. It's best when this therapist does not argue with you as to whether or not MCS is a mental condition, but instead simply helps you learn to live your life and still be contented — as opposed to starting behavioral therapy to tackle your so-called "chemophobia," which MCS is not. (Although of course it's up to you to choose among these approaches.) If you ask your doctor or therapist to read *Part I* of this book, it may have a positive impact on their attitude toward you.

182. Detoxification

In case of a slowed or impaired detoxification system, it's important to look for other ways to detoxify. With the help of an MCS-safe sauna, food supplements that enable detoxification and physical exercise, it's possible to improve. Seek help from a specialist who can guide you in this and who is informed of your situation (see *question 15* and *entry 298*. In Dr. Rea's book (see *entry 328*), you can find information about a good approach to detoxification.

Also see *entries 247* and *249* and www. the-abc-of-mcs.com under "Sauna."

Warning: Be very careful with fast and drastic approaches. You should first seek proper supervision and acquire the necessary knowledge. Detoxifying too quickly can even be harmful, because the chemical substances that are released can't properly be removed and instead circulate throughout your body. These circulating chemical substances can then cause damage and actually give you more problems.

183. Diet

See *entry 248.*

184. Dish detergent

There are various dish detergents for hand and machine washing which are suitable for MCS patients. Regular dish detergents contain too many synthetic chemicals and are not advisable. In natural and organic stores as well as online stores you can find healthy alternatives. It's just a matter of looking around and trying out different products to see which brands and detergents you can tolerate. When possible, choose a product that is as close to all-natural as you can find, in order to minimize the burden of chemical substances in your home and life as much as possible.

PRODUCTS TO TRY OUT

Dish detergent (hand): www.lesstoxic guide.ca/index.asp?fetch=household#dish

Dish detergent (machine) www.less toxicguide.ca/index.asp?fetch=househo ld#dish2

Or go to the several links mentioned in *Part VI* which sell MCS products.

TIP

You can also make your own dish detergent and cleaning solution using things such as lemon, salt, baking soda, borax and vinegar. See *entry 174.*

185. Doctor visits

Seeing a mainstream doctor who does not have knowledge of MCS can be a very exhausting and sometimes frustrating process. Whether or not your doctor is familiar with and acknowledges MCS depends in large part on his particular field of interest. The human body is still a very complex system, which often makes it difficult to correctly pinpoint the cause of many problems. Many times doctors thus try to find a solution by fighting the symptoms. When this doesn't help, some doctors automatically start looking for an answer in the psychological field, especially with MCS.

Once such a diagnosis has been entered into your medical files, you won't easily get it removed and you can take it for granted that future "vague ailments" may also be interpreted as signs of a mental problem. This, of course, doesn't get you anywhere.

Many physicians who take MCS seriously are occupational and environmental health specialists. Of course it is always good to inform your mainstream doctor about MCS if your doctor does not seem to know much about it. Some mainstream doctors really do care and are open to learning new things and gaining new insights.

When visiting a mainstream doctor, do not let his or her lack of knowledge and understanding affect your sense of self-esteem.

186. Dry cleaning

Most dry cleaners treat clothes and other items using chemicals; this is thus not recommended for MCS patients. If you must make use of them, then hang up the cleared item for at least a week outside or in front of an open window so that it may gas out.

There are also dry cleaners that work without harmful chemicals; see *entry 350.*

187. Dryer

If you have to purchase a new clothes dryer, make sure to first let it run in another room or in a shed before bringing it into your home. It's probably better to buy an air dryer whereby the air is taken outside through a flexible tube, as opposed to a condensation dryer, whereby the air is blown into the room. Especially with a new machine that has not been gassed out, it's best to prevent the chemical vapors released when the dryer runs from being blown into your home.

188. Ecological living community

Developing ecological living communities for MCS patients is a great idea. These are communities like some in Arizona and New Mexico where cars, perfumes, barbecues and all kinds of sickmaking substances and chemicals are forbidden. Many countries have not gotten this far, but once more patients fall ill, more living ecological living communities will no doubt follow. Also see *entry 192.*

FOR SOME EXAMPLES, SEE

Seagonville Ecology Housing (only for patients of www.ehcd.com)
www.ehcd.com/websteen/seagoville.htm

Quail Haven MCS Housing (Arizona):

http://madelinx.tripod.com
http://dianeensign.tripod.com/index.html

FOR MORE RESOURCES, GO TO

http://mcs-america.org/EnvironmentalIllnessMCSSupportandReosurces.htm

189. Electro smog

If you react sensitively to radiation from digital enhanced cordless telecommunications (DECT) phones, video screens, electricity from waterbeds, chairs, and so forth, there are various ways to lessen electro smog or to protect yourself against it. See *Part VI* for several websites that can help you along in this subject. Interesting links are also listed on www.the-abc-of-mcs.com under "Electro smog."

SOME TIPS ABOUT PHONE CALLS

Having problems holding a cell phone up to your ear? Use a Mockia or Pokia, a separate radiation-free handset which you can plug into your cell phone! It's really neat and makes for a much more pleasant phone call. The handset may have to be gassed out. Available through www.mockia.com/store.html.

THERE ARE MULTIPLE SOLUTIONS
TO THE RADIATION OR GASES
COMING FROM COMPUTERS

• Put the PC in a different room and run the cables through wall to the video monitor.

• Always go with a flat screen monitor (LCD or TFT); these give off very little radiation.

• For an interesting example of a far-reaching adjustment regarding the computer, visit: www.asilo.com/aztap1. This page discusses an electrical engineer's work developing low-emissions computers.

• Another informative and interesting site concerning the computer is www.greenmachineshop.com/html/gassing-out.html.

190. Electronic candles

A good alternative to burning candles is electronic candles — really LED lights that run on rechargeable batteries. The lights flicker just like normal candles and, because they're encased in a clouded glass holder, they still provide something like the cozy atmosphere of real candles. See also *entry 167.*

191. Electronic devices and machines

New devices should always be gassed out before use for a long time. The gases that are released by a new computer or television, for example, can make you very sick (due, among other things, to the brominated flame retardant substances which these devices often contain nowadays). A computer or a television off-gasses when turned on and exposed to heat; for this reason it's good to let it run in another room, using a time switch if necessary. If you just leave the television in its box in the attic for a year, you may still have trouble with gases when the device heats up for the first time. For more information on brominated flame retardants, search on www.greenpeace.org/usa.

These days, there are devices available that allow you to remotely control all your electronics, such as a DVD player, video recorder, TV, tuner and so on. This lets you put all your new sound and video devices in a different room, which you can then control with this remote control, through a so-called "eye." You'll have fewer problems associated with the gases from these devices, while still being able to immediately enjoy their use. An example of such an infrared eye is the 291 series IR receiver by Xantech (for an example and more information, see these links: www.hometech. com/infrared/rcvrs.html#XA-29110 and www.xantech.com/manuals/29110.pdf).

Never let your television gas out at someone else's house, unless there is no other way, because the television can absorb substances such as perfume or smoke from the room it's in. When the TV heats up (when you turn it on), it will then give off these substances for a long time! Gassing out a TV can take months, even if it's being run eight hours per day in a different room. For some devices, such as a vacuum cleaner, it's a good idea to keep a backup. When your old one breaks, at least you'll have a new one ready to go, already gassed out in your "gassing-out room." This saves you from having to deal with gases being released from the hose or motor when you use a new vacuum. A device

like a vacuum cleaner just can't be missed, as it's needed every day, which is why you want to keep a backup ready to go. For tips about the dryer, see *entry 187.*

192. Emigration

In some cases, for example when you can no longer tolerate the outside air, emigrating to a different country or moving to an other state could be the solution. But make no mistake, you will encounter stress and difficulties: tons of organizing and arranging, giving up your "safe" home, the journey, new home, new life, insurance, work, and so forth.

You should also realize that it's no longer 100 percent safe anywhere in the world. You will find chemical substances, people smoking, fires and stoves just about everywhere. Finding a place that is 100 percent safe is thus really a utopian ideal.

The less populated an area is, the better chance you have of encountering clean land, clean air and a better environment, but you could still have problems from things like forest fires or industrial activity in the area or even in a neighboring country or area. Rural areas may also have many farmers making frequent use of pesticides. And the more rural a place gets, the more limited the available provisions are. There won't be a natural foods store and probably no grocery delivery service or any other aid. If you live in a very urban or industrial area with heavy air pollution, you might first want to think about moving to a more rural area to find some cleaner air (although in these places, depending on the state and country, you may find stoves and fireplaces in the winter as well).

Should you still want to move, inform yourself very well, and do realize that social isolation is often a necessity even in "clean" places, since synthetic cleaning products and perfumes have been integrated into almost all societies. One option is to look for an ecological/natural living community or to live in an MCS community like the ones in Arizona and New Mexico. Canada also has some options in this regard. But don't just think that it's an easy thing to move into these places or that you'll be welcomed with open arms, because in New Mexico, for example, many MCS patients are still looking for safe, affordable housing. So there, too — especially if you are of modest financial means — you'll run into the usual MCS housing problem.

If you are making plans in this direction, it's advisable that you become a member of the Canadian and American online MCS networks so that you can find and receive more information on the subject. See *Part VI* for several groups or www.the-abc-of-mcs.com under "Groups."

CHECK OUT THESE
LINKS AS WELL

No Safe Haven
People With Multiple Chemical Sensitivity Are Becoming the New Homeless: www.emagazine.com/view/?1003
Yahoo group about short-term and long-term housing for people with MCS http://health.groups.yahoo.com/group/mcssafeshelterusa
www.planetthrive.com/members/PD

Fs/Safer%20Construction%20Tips%20read%20only.pdf

193. Environmental health centers

See *question 15* and *entry 298* and see *Part VI.*

194. Exercise

Outdoor exercise is almost no longer possible if you have MCS: jogging on the street is not recommended because of car exhaust and swimming in pools is inadvisable due to the chlorine in the water. Indoor sports expose you to the laundry products and shampoos of others, and with team sports you'll have to deal with physical contact. Exercising while wearing a mask is almost impossible due to the lack of oxygen that can quickly arise, although there are special breathing masks for running and walking. Find out about these at www.respro.com/products/sports-leisure/running-walking/aero_mask.

But daily exercise is most definitely still necessary, especially if you're always at home. Purchasing a treadmill or a home trainer is a good investment in your health. And of course exercising outdoors in natural areas — such as jogging or hiking on the beach or in the forest — is still doable as long as you're not dealing with others or teammates.

195. Faith

Many people find strength in faith, whether or not they follow any specific religion or group. Sharing spiritual or religious convictions often helps MCS patients, even if it's a problem for MCS patients to leave the home and go to church or a meeting. In the United States, special websites and chemical-free services for MCS patients have been established, and newsletters are circulated. Some churches in the US already run a completely scent-free program. Also see *entry 374*, and find some inspiring examples at these sites: www. aromaofchrist.com; http://health.grou ps.yahoo.com/group/CMCS-EI; www. sharecareprayer.org.

196. Fever

Fever can be your body's reaction to too many toxic substances in the blood, but it can also be a consequence of an infection somewhere in the body. Fevers above 104°F can even be dangerous. In case of a persistent or high fever you should certainly consult your doctor. Ask your doctor whether a course of antibiotics is absolutely necessary, since this can cause your MCS situation to deteriorate considerably. If your fever is not severe, perhaps you can first try to find a cure using natural products or other safe alternatives. Also see *entry 201*.

197. Fireplaces

See *entry 291*.

198. Fireworks

Celebrating the Fourth of July, New Year's Eve, or other holidays traditionally involving fireworks is no longer fun for most MCS patients (or for those with asthma and respiratory problems). You'll just have to stay inside on those days and hermetically seal all doors and windows when fireworks are being set off. A good air purifier (see *entry 144*) is a must in order to get through these holidays without consequences.

199. Floor covering

New carpets, laminate, parquet, vinyl, and so on are not suitable for MCS patients, because the varnishes, glues, synthetic substances, formaldehyde and other chemical substances can cause severe problems. Gassing out these chemicals can take months if not years. It's therefore best to play it safe and go with materials that are less harmful, such as organically produced cotton. An untreated hardwood floor or other hard floor coverings, like stone, ceramic or porcelain tile, are also good options. Make sure you do not react to the specific wood by first testing a sample thoroughly!

If you're looking for safe floor covering, it's wise to start gathering information on the various ecological and safe options. Keep in mind that "green products" are not necessarily safe for MCS patients. See also http://users.lmi.net/ wilworks/ehnlinx/f.htm#Flooring, or www.the-abc-of-mcs.com under "Living," where you can find links to sites that could help you (for example a very helpful document by Planet Thrive, "Safer Construction Tips for the Environmentally Sensitive").

Of course, after thoroughly researching the options, you will first take home a large piece of the relevant material and test it by placing it somewhere near you. You will also make sure that the installation of your natural floor covering will not require glues and/or will occur in an ecologically responsible manner.

If your floor is covered with something that is making you sick, there is only one solution: get it out! (or at least make sure you do not have to be in that particular room for a long time) It should go without saying that you will have others do it for you and not start tearing out the floor covering yourself.

200. Flowers

Do not put flowers in your home that have come from a mainstream garden center or any place like that, because these tend to have been sprayed repeatedly with pesticides. Stick with flowers from your yard or buy organically produced flowers. Some examples about organic flowers are found at: www.local harvest.org/organic-flowers.jsp and www. ecobusinesslinks.com/organic_flowers. htm.

201. Flu-like symptoms

This is a pretty common symptom of MCS, although this phenomenon can arise due to small infections in the respiratory system, but also in other places in the body, without necessarily giving you a high fever. It's important to prevent further exposures and to give your body time to recover. Unbalanced intestinal bacteria can also cause flu-like symptoms. Consult your general practi-

tioner first. It's also a good idea to go to an environmental health specialist or therapist for testing to see if there aren't other causes underlying your symptoms.

202. Food

See *entry 248.*

203. Food supplements

Supplements are not necessarily harmless products. Too much of anything can cause severe medical problems. If you choose to take supplements, have yourself supervised by an expert! See also *entry 249.*

204. Formaldehyde

Formaldehyde is found in construction materials such as particle board and triplex, textiles, floor covering, furniture, soft plastic, paper, paint, glues, household products, ink, and tobacco smoke, and can cause serious problems for MCS patients. For information about formaldehyde, see www.allergybuyerscl ub.com/learning/montanaformaldehyde. html.

According to research from Japan tea bags (black and green tea) can be used to help absorb formaldehyde gases in a new home. But it's better, of course, to avoid all materials that contain formaldehyde, rather than having to deal with tea bags afterwards! See: www.newscientist.com/ article/mg16722481.700-tea-versus-toxi ns.html. The air purifier IQair Multi-gas also can remove formaldehyde (see *entry 144*).

SOURCES

B.A. Sorg, et al., "Exposure to Repeated Low-Level Formaldehyde in Rats Increases Basal Corticosterone Levels and Enhances the Corticosterone Response to Subsequent Formaldehyde." *Brain Research* April 20, 2001; 898(2):31420. www.ncbi.nlm.nih.gov/pubmed/11306018?dopt=AbstractPlus.

D.K. Sari, et al., "Effect of Prolonged Exposure to Low Concentrations of Formaldehyde on the Corticotropin-Releasing Hormone Neurons in the Hypothalamus and Adrenocorticotropic Hormone Cells in the Pituitary Gland in Female Mice." *Brain Research* July 2, 2004; 1013(1): 10716. www.ncbi.nlm.nih.gov/pubmed/15196973?dopt=AbstractPlus.

205. Forums

An online forum is a group of people who exchange all kinds of tips and experiences with each other through the Internet. This can very useful if you need information on certain issues or are looking for an address or a product that you can tolerate. There are many online forum groups all over the world. See *Part VI* for several links, or go to www.the-abc-of-mcs.com under "Groups."

206. Frontal lobe sinus infections

See *entry 286*.

207. Furniture

As with all new materials, few new furniture items are immediately safe for use, since chemical substances and synthetic materials are used in the production of furniture. It's a matter of gassing things out or finding furniture produced in an environmentally responsible way.

Information about safer furniture can be found at: www.furnature.com and www.nontoxic.com.

208. Gloves

To prevent chemical substances from getting on your hands, it's a good idea to wear gloves. There are various options, such as latex and nitrile. Yet nitrile rubber is a synthetic product that is made using materials derived from crude oil that can cause reactions in an MCS patient. Natural rubber (latex) is extracted from the rubber tree and is thus in most cases safer for MCS patients, but not suitable for those with an allergy to latex. If, for example, your partner works or comes into contact with certain substances outside of the home and wants to come inside safely, it would be good for him or her to seek protection in the form of nitrile or latex. Nitrile offers better protection against chemical substances than latex. If you purchase new rubber, latex or latex-free gloves for doing household chores, let them off-gas outside (under an awning or in a shed) for some time before using them, until you are sure you can use them without having a reaction.

209. Glue

A good alternative to synthetic glue is a natural glue. Using natural glue is not, however, a guarantee that you can tolerate it. If you can, leave gluing to others, and let the glued item gas out before bringing it into your safe living space. If you'd like to work with these materials yourself, make sure you test them beforehand and, just to be sure, wear protection if you're not sure yet whether or not you react to the glue. In general all kinds of glue can be gassed out pretty well; but do make sure the item in question can gas out safely after it has been glued.

An example of 100 percent natural glue is Auro Contact Glue. See: www. metaefficient.com/adhesives-caulks-and-sealants/auro-contact-glue-100-natural.html.

210. Groups

See *entry 205* and *Part VI.*

211. Hair salon

At the hair salon many products are used that can make an MCS patient sick. For this reason, ask the hairdresser to come to your home and choose a product that is as safe as possible for you, or go to a hairdresser who uses only natural products. Yet in the latter case you still can't be sure that the environment there is safe for you, given the laundry detergents and perfumes possibly used by the other customers and the staff.

If you wear your hair at an even length and wear a ponytail, it can easily be cut by a partner, friend or family member. Nobody will notice that it might be a bit uneven. If you have (very) short hair you could just use hair clippers.

Some examples of organic hair salons can be seen at: http://hair.lovetoknow. com/Aveda_Organic_Hair_Salon, www. johnmasters.com/salon.htm, and www. ecocolors.net.

212. Hangover

A reaction to a chemical irritant can feel much like the hangover from excessive consumption of alcohol. It's even possible for somebody to first experience a pleasant "up" from certain substances, followed by a "down" (hangover). The withdrawal symptoms, which have been described by Dr. Rea, can be quite intense and often indicate poisoning and detoxification. After the liver has processed the substances, these symptoms tend to disappear.

213. Happiness

"Happiness comes from the soul within" may be a cliché, but it's certainly a truthful statement. You yourself control a large portion of your happiness, no matter how bad the circumstances of your life may be. If you feel unhappy and consider yourself a victim of your disease, it's good to keep searching for ways to become happier. Despite your tough situation, try to make something of your life. You can either keep mourning for that which you lost or focus on new perspectives according to your situation.

Given the fact that chemical substances can make you depressed (through the influence these substances exert on the brain), the consistent avoidance of chemical substances is a big step forward on the path to happiness! It's easier to feel contented in a healthy body. Allow yourself to be inspired by good spiritual books on this subject and, for example, seek out TV programs or movies that portray people who, despite being considerably handicapped or even severely disfigured, are still happy. Or speak to fellow MCS patients and ask them what they do to maintain happiness.

Find new goals and perspectives in your life: writing, making music, learning languages, adopting new hobbies that are easy to do within the home, and so on. Lying in bed or on the couch will quickly turn you into an uninspired, discontented person. Playing the hand you're dealt will allow you to keep on moving forward and enjoy the things that come to you on your path, even if your life is not what you had imagined it to be. This is usually the biggest shock that you have to come to terms with. Also see *Part II: The Personal Situation* for more on this subject.

214. Helmet

See *entry 274*.

215. Homeopathic medicines

Homeopathic medicines can have a good supportive role, but you still need to determine what products you can tolerate. Alcohol, for example, which is the basis for many homeopathic liquid drops, could induce a negative reaction. See this website for good regular information on homeopathic medicines: www.ritecare.com/homeopathic/guide_general.asp. Consult a good therapist who is knowledgeable about MCS.

216. Hospitals

If you have to go into a hospital, prepare yourself very thoroughly in order to get through this period as safely as possible. The following are a number of tips:

• First of all, if you are diagnosed with MCS, bring a letter from your environmental health specialist, or ask him or her to write one for the hospital explaining the adjustments necessary for your situation.

• Make sure you get treated by doctors and nurses who are fragrance-free, or at least do not wear perfume or aftershave.

• Protect yourself as much as possible using respiratory protection (see *entry 274*).

• Perhaps ask for a room to yourself in the hospital, which, if at all possible, has been cleaned using only baking soda (sodium bicarbonate).

• If permitted, bring your own bedding, soap and towels.

• Bring your own quality air purifier which you can place right beside your bed.

• If anesthesia will come into play, ask for an anesthetic that does not have to be inhaled, since gas anesthetics can make you more ill.

• Drink your own purified water as much as possible.

• Do not allow open containers of chemicals in your room.

• When you need oxygen, use a ceramic mask instead of plastic.

• Try to keep your stay in the hospital as short as possible and to have any possible checkups conducted at your home. Ask if your general practitioner can come by to do it. You could also just go back to the hospital each day for the checkups. Consult your doctor about the possibilities.

These suggestions are compiled with a severe MCS patient in mind. Those with chemical sensitivity who are able to lead relatively normal lives will no doubt need to take fewer precautions.

For more considerations and suggestions for an MCS-adjusted hospital stay or an adjusted visit, go to *entry 360* or to: www.ctaz.com/~bhima/hospital.htm, www.immuneweb.org/articles/anesthetics.html, or www.mcscanadian.org/hospital.html.

217. Hotels

Staying in hotels is not easy for MCS patients, due to the cleaning products that are used and the disinfecting synthetic laundry products used for the sheets and towels. Smoking is also a problem. Depending on the state or country, guests may be allowed to smoke indoors. There is a special hotel designed for MCS patients in Florida: www.thenaturalplace.com. For more links on traveling with MCS, go to www.the-abc-of-mcs.com under "Traveling."

Also see *entry 301.*

218. Housing

Living anywhere safely is very difficult for MCS patients. If you have to move, definitely research the location you want to move to. Look out for industry, lots of traffic, and other factors. Living in urban or industrial areas is not ideal for MCS patients, who are better off choosing rural or coastal locations. Even then you're not guaranteed an entirely safe location, because everywhere in the country people are stoking stoves and furnaces that pollute the outside air, farmers are using pesticides, and so on, so prepare yourself adequately in this regard. Even if you opt for an ecological house, which of course is much better than a "normal" new housing development, you still will have to deal with your surrounding environment! No matter where you are, it's always important to make your house as safe as possible for you and to ensure constant air purification. See Chapter 2 for more information.

At *entry 192*, concerning moving to another country or state, you will find several interesting links on the subject of housing. Also see: www.the-abc-of-mcs.com under "Living."

219. Hyperventilation

MCS is not a form of hyperventilation or a panic response. Just as some people with asthma can hyperventilate or panic when exposed to a harmful substance, the same can occur in some people with MCS.

In case you have been diagnosed with hyperventilation syndrome or you often hyperventilate, you can ask your doctor for breathing and relaxation exercises to bring it under control. Hyperventilation can arise because of improper breathing (overbreathing) caused by shortness of breath, but it can also arise as a reaction to anxiety and stress. Be sure to keep possible panic reactions to certain scents under control, because you don't necessarily face severe reactions to every scent. Always keep adequate protection on hand, so that you can step outside feeling more at ease and won't panic so easily when something crops up. This will have a favorable effect upon any possible hyperventilation attack. Also see *entries 18* and *19*.

Reiki has a very relaxing and regulating effect in case of hyperventilation (also see *entry 272* and www.het-abc-van-reiki.nl/en/). Especially in combination with conscious stomach breathing, during which you hold your hands on your stomach, it has a very calming effect. Make sure you bring down your breathing and let it normalize.

For further information, visit www.e medicinehealth.com/hyperventilation/ar ticle_em.htm and www.relaxandbrea the.net.

220. Infections

See *entries 196, 201* and *286*.

221. Ink

Printer ink can induce a reaction. It's best to put the printer in a room with open windows which you don't have to enter. You can also let printed items (including photos) air out and then place them in a large off-gassed plastic storage bag with zipper. Purchasing a reading box (see *entry 271*) is a way to avoid getting sick from the ink on books or magazines. Many newspapers and mag-azines can nowadays be found online. Avoid opening the mail without respiratory protection and, for writing, use a pencil instead of a pen or a marker.

222. Inner peace

Discovering that you have MCS usually marks the start of a quest for healing and recognition. Yet most of the time you'll find you simply won't receive recognition for your illness due to the lack of knowledge about the disease, including among conventional doctors and other caregivers. Your best bet is to visit experts on this environmental illness, from whom you can get understanding, support and the proper knowledge.

While you are researching the opportunities for betterment with regard to your home, your life and the condition of your health, it is possible to achieve a certain form of inner peace. Accepting the fact that your life isn't perfect (but also doesn't have to be perfect) is a first step towards inner peace. We can't have everything, and some people will simply face more obstacles on their path than others. If you use these obstacles to grow within and become a stronger and more beautiful person, you will find more inner peace than if you keep looking back to what could have been. Those kinds of thoughts can cause a great deal of anxiety. Learning that you can choose how you view your life will only increase your chances of achieving inner peace. You could also undertake various activities to augment your inner peace, such as meditating (see *entry 238*), Reiki (see *entry 272*) and reading inspiring books (see *entry 340*). Also see *entry 213*.

223. Insect Repellents

Choose an all-natural anti-mosquito product, such as the Herbal Insect Repellent from Real Purity (http://realpurity.com) or a different product that can be easily tolerated, but avoid all chemical creams and spray cans. It is very risky to keep using such products with regard to the possible deterioration of your situation. If you're able to tolerate essential oils, tea tree oil is also a good substance to ward off mosquitoes and other biting insects. It also helps treat the itch and the swelling when you've already been bitten. Use organic tea tree oil (see *entry 297*). Avoid cheaper (often synthetic) essential oils, which can cause reactions in those with sensitivities. Do not use a mosquito net that has been treated with an insecticide.

224. Insecticides/Pesticides

It should go without saying that an MCS patient should never come into contact with insecticides or pesticides. Use a mosquito net and window screens. Work with organic products or have someone else do the work for you outside, but never use harmful chemicals within your home. Also see *entry 372.*

It's important to create as much of a balance in your garden as possible, such that you don't have to use insecticides in the first place. Insects are part of nature, which includes the garden, and if they're not overwhelming your yard, you ought to just leave them alone. Over time they leave on their own accord (or get eaten by birds).

TIPS FOR WEEDING BETWEEN TILES

Either remove weeds by hand (a new hobby for once you've gone into isolation!), use vinegar or use a propane-fired weed torch, which kills weeds with heat. Make sure you protect yourself from the propane.

Here are some links to less harmful nontoxic pest control. They are not specifically made for MCS patients, so be careful. www.maskedflowerimages.com/pestcontrol.html, www.maskedflowerimages.com/nontoxicpestcontrol.htm, www.safesolutionsinc.com. See also Steve Tvedten's very informative website about free nontoxic pest control: www.thebestcontrol.com.

225. Instructions, list of

Below you will find an example of a thorough list of instructions for visitors to your home. This list is, of course, adjustable according to the degree to which changes are necessary, depending on the severity of your MCS.

Dear ———,

How wonderful that you'd like to come visit me and how great that you're willing to do anything you can to make this visit be as safe as possible for me, and take extensive precautionary measures. What follows is a list of instructions, as promised:

• Wash *all* the clothing (including underwear, socks, jeans, sweater, etc.) you will be wearing separately in the washing machine, at least three times as long as usual and as hot as possible, using my laundry detergent and some baking soda (which I'll give you).

• Make sure all the remaining detergent in the detergent loader is first removed.

• With strongly perfumed/scented clothing it's recommended to first soak it in water with a cup of isopropyl alcohol and then to wash it a number of times using my detergent and baking soda.

- Let your clothes dry outside or in the attic (not in the bathroom), rather than the dryer, to minimize the chance that residual perfume will get on them.
- Keep these safe clothes separate from your normal clothes until your visit. Don't store them in new plastic, but if you'd like to wrap them, use aluminum foil. Once you've created a safe set of clothing, it's perhaps a good idea to always keep these separate, reserved for these visits. You could also store this set of clothes at my house.
- Do not wear new clothing or clothing which has just come from the dry cleaner. Let them air out for a week in front of an open window or outside under an awning.
- Do not wear an unsafe jacket, but rather a properly washed vest or fleece sweater.
- For at least two days before your visit, wash your hair and yourself using the body shampoo (which I'll provide you with) and dry yourself with a towel which was washed using my detergent.
- Please don't apply anything to yourself or your hair which did not come from me (or with my recommendation), not even a tiny bit!
- I'll also be giving you soap and shampoo and perfume-free deodorant (unless you already have perfume-free toiletries: please check with me first).
- If you need gel or hair spray, please let me know and I'll give you these things as well.
- On the way to my house, don't stop by even briefly at any other places, especially not places where people are smoking or where there are many chemical substances (such as perfume, paint, air fresheners, cleaning products, etc.).
- Don't smoke any more after you've made yourself completely safe to come visit me.
- I'd rather you didn't wear lipstick; it can off-gas scents and might get on my face in the course of warm greeting kisses; other makeup, such as eye shadow or mascara, can be used without problems.
- Only use the foundation or day cream that you receive from me.
- Do not polish your nails on the day of the visit (the day before is no problem).
- Don't go to the hair salon and get a perm or hair dye right before the visit.
- Do not wear recently polished shoes, new shoes or shoes recently treated with any kind of a spray can.

- If you have one, remove the air freshener from your car and air your car out before you drive to my house.
- Do not bring flowers or plants, unless they are organic or meant for the yard. Your visit is far more important to me than a gift!

I hope this won't be too much for you! Of course I'm willing to help by providing further explanation where necessary. If there are other things that you're unsure about and/or that aren't on this list, please discuss these with me beforehand. If you'd like to look up some information yourself, visit www.the-abc-of-mcs.com.

See you soon! It's so kind of you to do all this to be able to visit me!

Love,

———

INSTRUCTIONS FOR YOURSELF
TO KEEP THE VISIT AS SAFE
AS POSSIBLE FOR YOU

Make sure you have your air purifier running on high and that you place Tyvek (see *entry 306*) over your couch, and on top of this a couch cover. This prevents any residual substances on the clothes of your visitor(s) from staying on your couch and giving you problems later on. Before or during the visit air the room out thoroughly. If necessary, use a fan to get the remaining gases out of your home as quickly as possible. During the visit you can protect yourself with the many options that exist in this regard. See *entry 274.*

226. Instructions for your partner

Because partners tend to leave the house quite often, it's important that they adhere to certain instructions upon coming back inside. It's good to make agreements with each other in order to make your partner's homecoming as safe as possible for you. Here are a few suggestions for severe MCS patients.

Set aside a room which you don't have to enter where your partner can change out of and hang the clothes worn outside. Ideally, he or she won't have to walk through the room that you're in at the time with unsafe clothing on. Your partner could even undress in a hallway or a shed if a bathrobe is left there for him or her to put on. If he or she needs to walk through the safe room (for instance on the way to the bathroom to shower and change into safe indoor clothing), make sure he or she wears this bathrobe and a towel over his or her head. Whenever your partner has been elsewhere, no matter the circumstances, it's good for him or her to shower or at least wash the hair and face. In all cases he or she should change into a special set of safe home clothing.

227. Internet

A great deal of information is available on the Internet. The ABCs of MCS (www.the-abc-of-mcs.com) is a good place to start learning about the subject. If you've made useful discoveries online which would be interesting for this site, please write to webmaster@het-abc-van-mcs.nl.

Indeed, the Internet is also exquisitely suited for maintaining many contacts and discovering new people (fellow patients?) and things (about MCS?). It's also a "super store" for all kinds of products, which allows you to shop indoors.

228. Ionizer, portable

See *entry 144*.

229. IQair

See *entry 144*.

230. Laundry detergents

There are various laundry products available to MCS patients. Here, too, you should test things to see which products work for you. One person might do just fine with the brands Ecover and Seventh Generation, while other people will have to keep looking for other suitable detergents. The perfume-free laundry products from supermarkets are usually not chemical-free and are thus best avoided. In natural stores and various online shops you can find many different organic laundry detergents which are suitable for MCS patients. See www.the-abc-of-mcs.com under "Products (Online)," or see *Part VI* for many addresses.

TIPS

• The soap nut (sapindus) is an organic laundry detergent, originally from India and Nepal. The shell of the soap nut contains a sticky substance called saponin, which has the same properties as normal soap. When the nutshells come into contact with water, it creates a mild soap solution. See http://sapindus.org and www.maggiespureland.com. Nowadays these soap nuts are also available in liquid form; see www.maggies pureland.com/liquid.html.

• Very sensitive MCS patients sometimes use only baking soda as a laundry detergent; for more information on this product, see *entry 154*.

• Another alternative for laundry detergent is to use washing soda. This product is sold in the detergent aisle of most supermarkets. Make sure you choose the scent-free variant. Health food stores sometimes sell pure washing soda as well.

231. Leather

Leather undergoes many chemical treatments before it can become a shoe, jacket or couch, and new items are thus not safe for an MCS patient. You can either choose secondhand leather items or allow new leather products to gas out for quite a long time.

232. Leisure and entertainment

If you can no longer go outdoors, it's still very important to entertain yourself with something. Find hobbies that are still possible or pick up the activities that you never got around to but always wanted to do, which you'll have all the time in the world for now. There is more out there than you think. It's often just a matter of realigning your perspectives and learning to look for that which you can still do. Also see *Part II: The Personal Situation* and *Part III: The Voices of Others*.

233. Magazines

See *entry 221*.

234. Masks

See *entry 274*.

235. Materials

In general no new material is initially safe for MCS patients. Learn as much as you can about using natural and organic materials, because these usually can be used immediately. Everything else, depending on the product, needs time to gas out. See also *entry 177*.

236. Mattresses

New synthetic mattresses tend to cause severe problems for MCS patients because they release chemical gases. You should search carefully for a mattress that's as safe as possible that you can tolerate. Choosing the right mattress is very dependent on the question of whether you're also allergic to its materials, or whether you can just go ahead and pick a mattress made of natural materials. "Natural" or "green" do not imply that the mattress is organic and do not mean it is necessarily safe for MCS patients.

So basically it's a choice between letting a new mattress gas out for an extensive period (this can take quite a long time), or purchasing a mattress made of natural/organic materials. See www.the-abc-of-mcs.com under "Living" for a several links to organic mattresses available in the United States, or go to *Part VI* for some online addresses.

Nowadays there are a number of mattresses available that are made of natural materials such as coconut, wool, cotton, natural rubber (latex), or horsehair, but they often are not organically produced. It's just a matter of conducting solid research!

Purchasing an old (secondhand) mattress is definitely not advisable. Such mattresses can be dusty or moist and can contain molds and old perfume particles.

237. Medicine

Medicines are made using synthetic materials, so it's possible that MCS patients will not tolerate them. In consultation with your doctor, try looking for safer/natural alternatives whenever possible. If you do have to use medicine, test it very carefully to start with. You may be able to pulverize a tablet and use just a tiny bit to see if you display any negative reactions. Then slowly build up the dosage, when possible. *Be sure to discuss this with your doctor*, since with some medications you actually can't do a slow buildup and have to immediately start with a high dosage, for example when eliminating bacteria and viruses.

238. Meditation

Meditation is absolutely recommended for MCS patients. Among other things, meditation can neutralize physical reactions to an exposure. It also has a deep impact on the spirit and helps foster inner peace. There are various options in this field, all of which can help and are easy to learn (at home). Visit the Internet for more information on the various methods.

One of the advisable and effective methods is Transcendental Meditation. See www.tm.org for more information. Also, using Reiki techniques (see *entry 272*) for meditation is a very relaxing and effective way of neutralizing physical reactions to chemicals and calming the body and soul.

Listed below is some information taken (with permission) from the translated manuscript of *The ABCs of Reiki*, specifically about meditation:

> Meditating is a way to give your mind peace, which in turn has a positive effect on your health, because a calm mind prevents your "teacup" (head) from overflowing! The Japanese very appropriately say: "You cannot fill up a full teacup."
>
> This means that if you regularly empty your "teacup" by meditating, you will create more space for creativity, inspiration and insight, which otherwise would not have had a chance, because your teacup is already filled to the brim. By connecting with the energy field in this way, you will also get more energy.
>
> There are many different forms of meditation these days. You can learn how to meditate relatively easily using the books that are available on the subject.
>
> In second degree Reiki you also learn how to meditate with symbols and mantras.
>
>   * * *
>
> At first you will probably feel as if you are wasting your time and that meditating is not really calming your mind. Meditating is a process that you "have" to go through.
>
> You do not normally learn this in one day; you can learn the technique in one day, but the notion of what it does to you will only come to you after a while.
>
> We usually want too much ... (for example a peaceful mind after just one meditation).
>
> When you start meditating, your first experience could be that you become aware of your restlessness — unfortunately, this could give you the idea that meditating makes you restless.
>
> In this case, the process is as follows:
>
> - awareness (restlessness)
> - perception (without resistance)
> - letting go (by accepting).

Obviously, the more you let go, the calmer the mind will become.

The effects of the meditation techniques of Transcendental Meditation have been scientifically researched. The effect of meditation on for example sick leave has been tested on a large scale. It turned out that there was a considerable drop in sick leave. Apart from that, people who meditated turned out to be healthier and happier. Above all, those who meditated appeared to have an influence on the energy field and therefore on their environment. There is proof that in areas where a lot of people meditate, there is for example less crime (see www.tm.org).

Other meditation techniques obviously also have an influence on your mind, the energy field and therefore your environment.

* * *

Some say that the only difference between meditating and praying is that during praying you talk and during meditating you listen.

Silence Is the Great Revelation
(Lao-Tse)

239. Mold

Having mold in your home is harmful to anyone's health and definitely so for MCS patients. Try to get rid of the mold in a natural way so you don't have to make use of harmful mold-killing products. At the very least, make use of less-toxic products and be sure to properly protect yourself when using them! Open the doors and windows as much as possible and wear a mask when applying the mold-removing product! It is best to identify the cause of the mold problem so you can prevent more mold from growing in your home. Regular ventilation is one of the most important ways to prevent mold.

TIPS

• Dab the moldy spots with a solution of vinegar or borax (also see *entry* *161)*, and leave it on for a while, so the liquid can soak.

• Hydrogen peroxide removes mold in a less toxic way. Make sure you are protecting yourself while using it. See www.mold-removal.biz/mold-removal-1101.htm.

• For various safer mold-killing products, see also: www.needs.com, www.aehf.com, and www.lesstoxicguide.ca.

240. Natural foods stores

If you're in isolation and can't go out to shop for groceries, you should ask around to see if there is a delivery service. Natural foods stores may have a delivery service, especially for sick people or shut-ins. See *Part VI* for more information.

241. Natural printing

A natural printer uses as many naturally based raw materials as possible. This does not necessarily mean that all MCS patients will immediately be able to tolerate the printed work, because in terms of their sensitivity everyone is different. But in any case these products are healthier and safer, because no harmful gases come from soy ink or recycled paper. For some examples, go to www.naturalprinting.net/index.html, www.naturalprinting.com, or www.naturalsourceprinting.com.

242. Neighbors

MCS patients tend to have trouble with their neighbors, due to things like the furnace or the barbecue grills that are fired up, the use of dryers, spraying pesticides, and so on. Neighbors can also cause problems for an MCS patient if they smoke in the yard or on the balcony. Your neighbors may or may not react with understanding and sympathy when you try explaining your situation. Many people simply can't put themselves in the shoes of an MCS patient, and they quickly dismiss you as a whiner. Try to stay as friendly and patient as possible. Hand them a brochure (see the back of this book) or a business card (see *entry 163*), to teach them about MCS. You might be able to get your neighbors to warn you (a phone call will suffice) when they're likely to cause you harm, for example by having a barbecue, or spraying pesticides in their yard. Expecting your neighbors to start using different laundry detergents or to stop smoking outside is usually asking too much. Only rarely will people be willing to go to such lengths to adjust to your needs.

243. Newspapers

You're better off not keeping newspapers in your safe living room due to the freshly printed ink which releases harmful gases. Instead, choose an online subscription or read the newspaper in a custom-fitted reading box (see *entry 271*). You could, of course, let the newspaper gas out first, but then you will always be reading old news! TV and the Internet can provide you with all the latest news.

244. Noise and Light

There are some MCS patients who react sensitively to noise and bright light. Here, as well, there is really just one remedy: avoid and protect as much as you can!

245. Nose filters

Nose filters are sort of like little cups made of synthetic materials, which you place in your nose. They can be of use in case of certain allergies, but most MCS patients can't tolerate the new materials. If you let the nose filters gas out very thoroughly, you may be able to start making use of this option. The mantra that you should always test to see if something works for you is applicable here as well. An MCS patient is most benefited by the activated charcoal filling (black filters), unless something like hay fever is also in play (white filters). The activated charcoal filters give some protection against chemical compounds but will not protect against toxic chemicals or fumes. Make sure you use better and heavier protection when faced with toxic chemicals or if your MCS is severe.

If you make use of nose filters, you should breathe through your nose as much as possible and keep your mouth closed, because chemical gases can also come in through your mouth. Nose filters (also called Better Breathers) are available at the pharmacy or online at www.betterbreathers.com and www.nosefilters.com/prod01.htm.

246. Notes

If, for example, there is a courier or deliveryman standing in front of your door and smoking a cigarette, ask him to first put out the cigarette before you open the door. (You often can converse through the closed door.) The same goes for a running engine, especially if the car or scooter is parked right in front of your door. Ask that they turn off the engine before you open the door. You can even write a note or make a nice sign with an explanation, which you can hang on your door and point to when you can't open up. It would be a shame if such a short, but nevertheless unsafe moment caused harmful substances to enter your home with their often inherent negative consequences.

If you have a lot of trouble with your short-term memory, it's useful to keep a notepad nearby on which you can immediately jot down ideas and such.

247. Oils

If the MCS patient can endure essential oils, then these are excellent substances with which to tackle skin problems. Make sure to research the given oil, because most oils cannot be applied to the skin in concentrated form — tea tree oil and lavender oil are a few exceptions to this, but just to be safe you should carefully test it.

Organic sunflower oil can be used to facilitate detoxification. The oil should be held the mouth for 15 to 20 minutes and then spit out (do not swallow it). Do this once or twice per day on an empty stomach. Also see the following link for more details: http://oilpulling.com.

248. Organic food

It's a good idea for MCS patients to completely switch to eating organic food and consuming organic drinks. This prevents many chemical substances from entering the body in the form of preservatives, color and taste additives, insecticides, and so on. Fruits and vegetables at grocery stores have often been sprayed and can either cause a negative physical reaction in MCS patients or otherwise add an unnecessary burden to their system. If you are lucky, there will be an organic foods store nearby where you can buy lots of tasty and healthy things. For meat eaters, there are also organic butchers. Just Google "organic meats" or ask your local health food store for possibilities or addresses.

See *Part VI* for more information about online organic food stores (as well as *entry 240*).

249. Orthomolecular substances

Orthomolecular substances (vitamins, minerals, etc.) are often used in treatments for all kinds of diseases. Many environmental doctors and therapists work with them. Unfortunately, these substances can contain synthetic additives such as sweeteners and other supplements, which when used in high dosage or frequently can cause a negative reaction or symptoms of poisoning, especially in cases of a slowed detoxification system. See *entry 27*.

Complementary food supplements can be an excellent adjunct to things like detoxification or in replenishing any possible shortages. But do take care to let yourself be guided by an expert who is informed about MCS and who is careful with the buildup and the dosage.

250. Out-gassing

Out-gassing, also in this book referred to as "airing out" or "off-gassing," is when new items release gases from the chemicals used in their production. New items are best allowed to gas out in a shed or storage area rather than in the main (chemical-free) house.

Devices, furniture, and things like clothes off-gas faster when subjected to heat. Devices and machines should be turned on in a well-ventilated room which you don't have to enter, hooked up to a time switch, if necessary. Plan for an off-gassing period of several months and in some cases even longer. Items which can get wet can be placed in a bath with baking soda. Storing, say, a book or other item in a box with a dish filled with baking soda on it can also help. Although an ionizer (see *entry 144*) is not suitable for MCS patients, it can be helpful for airing things out. However, the sun is the best out-gassing agent, so make good use of it during hot and sunny weather! In principle, everything can be gassed out; the necessary length of time just varies greatly between the different materials.

251. Out-gassing room

If your residence allows for it, designate a special "out-gassing" room in which to place new items which need time to gas out, anything from shoes to a television to a new couch. This room must be properly ventilated, and the MCS patient should never have to go inside it. Having such a room makes it easier to acquire new items without immediately getting sick from them. The only thing necessary is free space and patience (regarding the often very long time new products need to gas out).

252. Oxygen

After a harmful exposure, oxygen can help neutralize the bodily reaction. Also in case of shortness of breath, extra oxygen can provide relief. Be sure to purchase a ceramic MCS-oxygen mask (see *entry 171*) and a Tygon (see *entry 305*) tube, because the standard-issue mask and tube mostly are made of a soft synthetic material that needs to be gassed out for quite some time. See: www.emergencypax.com/oxygen, www.open-aire.com, and www.the-abc-of-mcs.com under "Water & Oxygen" and *entry 367*.

253. Ozone

Many MCS patients fall ill when there is too much ozone in the air, such as on smoggy days or in case of high summer temperatures. Devices that produce ozone, such as ionizers and printers, can be harmful to an MCS patient. See *Part VI* for several Internet links on air pollution.

254. Paint

"Normal" (synthetic) paint can usually create serious problems for MCS patients. It's thus best to look for natural paint, namely those kinds based in minerals or plants. Some paints contain a natural solvent and others use water for dilution. Even natural solvents can sometimes cause allergic reactions in sensitive people, so be careful. Natural paints based in water are without a doubt the safest for MCS patients. In any case, always first put some paint on a small out-gassed board and place it in your home to see if you react to it (perhaps even put the board next to your bed). Never paint your entire home or safe room in one go! First do the board test, then paint a wall, then paint a room and see if everything is still all right. Only then should you proceed with other rooms. See *Part VI* for several natural and organic solutions or go to www.the-abc-of-mcs.com under "Living."

255. Paper

Both for the environment and for yourself, it's best to use recycled paper as much as possible. Toilet paper from the natural products store is an acceptable substitute for the more "luxurious" non-recycled toilet paper which is chemically bleached and often colored and perfumed.

256. Parties

For most MCS patients, parties are no longer an option. You can host a chemical-free party yourself, in a smoke-free room in a restaurant, but be sure to invite only people who respect your situation; this increases the chance of a successful party. It's also wise to take a good air purifier with you and to have protective measures for breathing at your disposal. In order to enable your guests to make the necessary preparations, you can provide everyone with a list of instructions beforehand (see *entry 225*), along with a "sample packet" that includes laundry detergent, deodorant, soap, shampoo and other items such as hair spray. At the drugstore you can purchase small bottles and jars, such that you can use one large bottle to fill multiple small ones, to save on costs. You could even give the waiters at the restaurant this sample packet. Of course guests are not allowed to smoke, not even outside, because they'll unintentionally carry the chemicals from cigarette smoke inside with them on their clothing, hair and breath.

257. Partner

See *entry 226.*

258. PC

See *entries 189* and *191.*

259. Pendulum

See *entry 158.*

260. Perfume

Perfume and perfume-containing products should be avoided as much as possible, unless you're dealing with natural perfume (such as rose oil by the brand Dr. Hauschka, an example of a wonderful and 100 percent natural perfume). Products that mention "essential" oils might, due to the cost considerations on the part of the producer, be partially or completely synthetically made (do extensive research). Be aware of the fact that synthetic perfume scents are added to many products, such as personal care products, laundry detergents and clothes softeners. Indeed, it requires a great deal of adjustment to avoid all these kinds of products.

261. Perfume-free products

A number of perfume-free products are readily available in supermarkets. This does not mean that, for example, a perfume-free laundry detergent is also chemical-free. You won't easily find 100 percent natural/organic laundry and personal care products in the supermarket. For chemical-free products, it's best to go to a natural products store. You can also find various options online. Also see www.the-abc-of-mcs.com under "Products (online)" or go to *Part VI: Further Resources.*

262. Personal care products

It can be quite a challenge to find the right care products. MCS patients all react differently to the various options. You just have to try out different products and see which you can tolerate. Some stores offer small test samples and packages.

The best thing to do is to choose natural products made from plants and herbs, because products in the supermarket labeled as perfume-free may contain synthetic substances, and you can also get sick from something which has no scent (see *entry 19*).

An example of MCS-friendly care products that are 100 percent natural is the brand Real Purity. Even the glycerin used in this brand is natural, which is not the case with most products. These products have a natural, pleasant scent due to ingredients such as herbs, flower and fruit extracts, but they are not additionally scented with natural perfumes. Their inventory even includes good makeup, hair spray and gel. You can order items directly from Real Purity at www.realpurity.com.

Natural-products stores also have various organic and chemical-free products.

For more information see *Part VI: Further Resources* and www.the-abc-of-mcs.com under "Products (online)."

263. Pesticides/Insecticides

See *entry 224*.

264. Pets

Having MCS does not necessarily mean you can't keep pets, although there are MCS patients who also have allergies and thus can't tolerate having pets around them. MCS is not an allergy, so if you don't have problems with allergies, then pets can be welcome companions for those in isolation.

Having pets does require you to deal

with the problem of anti-flea products; chemical pipettes and flacons are not recommended, and an MCS patient can get quite sick when a cat or dog has recently been treated with such products.

Nowadays organic anti-flea products are available at pet stores, but this does not mean that every MCS patient can handle them. Be very careful with such products and always take preventative measures!

For online shops that sell organic flea products, Google "organic anti-flea products" or "organic flea control" and you will find many possibilities.

TIPS FOR FIGHTING FLEAS

• Wash your pet with an all-natural anti-flea shampoo such as tea tree shampoo.
• Vacuum the house thoroughly and keep it clean.
• Wash all baskets and blankets.
• Comb your pet's fur daily with a flea comb.

TIPS FOR PREVENTING FLEAS

• If you can tolerate essential oils, make a concoction of diluted tea tree, lavender, rosemary, lemon and eucalyptus oil; put this concoction (or even just diluted tea tree or eucalyptus oil) in a pump flacon and, during flea season, spray or sprinkle some of it on your dog every day. Always use a pure brand. The cat may not appreciate this treatment (and probably will want to lick it all up), so for this reason it might be better to just regularly use the flea comb.
• Keep the house very clean (vacuum thoroughly) and wash the pet's blankets and basket often.

• Giving your pet a garlic pill every day can also help prevent fleas.
• Make sure that your dog or cat won't easily contract fleas from other pets by barring other pets from your home. If you take your dog outside, watch that he or she doesn't come near other dogs, including in the vet's waiting room.
• You can find more information, among other places, through Google (search "natural flea control").

TIPS IN CASE OF TICKS

Check for ticks often and remove them immediately in the healthiest and safest way possible for the dog or cat: using tick tweezers or a nipper. This is a really easy process, and these tools are available everywhere (drug and pet stores, online, etc.).

TIPS FOR CAT LITTERS

Use organic or natural cat litter to prevent reactions to the chemicals used in regular cat litter. The following are two websites for natural and biodegradable cat litter that might be better suited for MCS patients: www.swheatscoop. com/home.html and www.elegantcatlitt er.com.

265. Physical exercise

MCS patients who have fallen into isolation, ought to still partake in physical exercise, by using a home trainer, treadmill, stepper machine, jumping rope or dancing. MCS patients can no longer go outside to walk, bike or jog (depending on the area in which you live), but fortunately there are plenty of options for indoor exercise.

266. Plants

Do not immediately put plants from garden centers in your room. First rinse them thoroughly and let them off-gas in a different room. Commercial flowers and plants are sprayed with chemical substances that could incite a negative reaction.

267. Printers

See *entries 221* and *253*.

268. Psychological support

Psychological support can be very helpful (also see *entry 181*). Due to the enormous changes of life with MCS, you may feel overwhelmed. It's nice to have someone entirely outside of your daily life with whom to get things off your chest and to ask for guidance in the coping process. Losing touch with your friends and family can also be so emotionally intense as to demand psychological help.

In case of exposure to chemical substances, it's also very important to try staying as relaxed as possible (stress hormones can burden your body even more) and have faith that you'll soon be okay again. Of course, you should always walk away immediately and protect yourself when something crops up, but panicking (stress!) does not help your (or your partner's) situation.

When necessary, seek help from somebody who can provide good spiritual assistance — and has respect and understanding for MCS — and be careful when using anti-depressants. Also see *entry 21* with regard to the therapies that have helped MCS patients, as well as those that didn't. In *Part II: The Personal Situation* you can read about my experiences with mental exercises and inner peace.

269. Radiation

See *entry 189*.

270. Reading

As an MCS patient, it's no longer an easy thing to just crack open a book and start reading. This makes most MCS patients sick. One solution is to use the reading box (see next question) or a gassed-out plastic sheath with a zipper. Books are often hard to gas out. You could take out books from the library (already used and aired out), but there is still no guarantee that you will tolerate these books. You could also read by laying a foil cover over the book, or using respiratory protection. Books printed on recycled paper and with soy ink cause fewer problems.

271. Reading box

Reading boxes made of Plexiglas are available (see below), which makes reading or browsing magazines possible for MCS patients. Plexiglas is tolerated well by most MCS patients and it doesn't absorb the scents of the magazines and the like. Another advantage is that Plexiglas is safer for use than actual glass (less

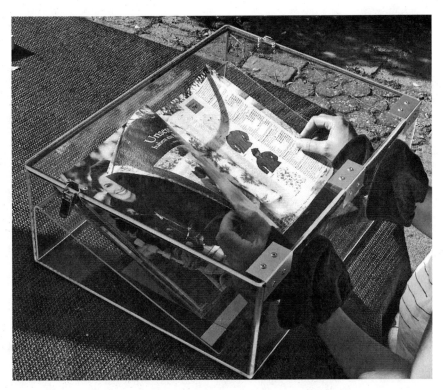

breakable) and is lighter. If the box has just come from the factory, it's a good idea to open it up outside (or in another room) and let it gas out for some time before using it, just to be sure.

To see two further examples of a reading box, go to http://mcsinfo.home stead.com/readingbox.html or http://au.geocities.com/dj_ludlow/mcs/read boxintro.pdf.

272. Reiki

Reiki is in most cases highly recommended for MCS patients. Reiki is a daily source of support with regard to inner peace, energy, neutralizing physical reactions, strengthening the immune system and, of course, detoxification.

Everyone can learn it, so as an MCS patient you can ensure that you're taught one-on-one by somebody who respects your situation and perhaps is even willing to come to your home. In any case, make sure that you find a teacher who is a good fit for you and does not insist on "curing" you before anything else. If you'd like to know more about Reiki, visit www.het-abc-van-reiki.nl/en.

Listed below are a number of questions and answers taken (with permission) from the translated manuscript of *The ABCs of Reiki.*

WHAT IS REIKI?

1. The Japanese word "Reiki" literally means "universal energy." "Rei" means "universal" and "Ki" means "energy."

2. Reiki is a method of working with energy.

When the word "Reiki" is used in this

book, it refers to the method of working with energy.

WHAT DOES REIKI DO?

Reiki is a method to take in energy from the energy field and to use it for yourself or others. At the physical level, each human has an immune system that has the ability to defend the body against foreign material, such as viruses and bacteria. This effort is fueled by energy, among other things. We know that if our immune system is functioning properly, we will be less susceptible to a cold or a virus and will recover more quickly if we do get ill.

At the mental level, energy increases your inner strength, which helps you feel good, which in turn has an effect on your health.

In other words, Reiki supports the self-healing ability of both the body and the mind.

HOW DOES REIKI WORK?

By nature (meaning from birth), everyone is able to take in energy from the energy field. This ability is being inhibited to a greater or lesser extent by various causes, as a result of which we are no longer able to take in enough energy. This is caused by our upbringing, culture, religion, the way we perceive nature and personal experiences. Reiki restores the ability to take in energy and thus helps you absorb energy better.

CAN REIKI BRING ABOUT SPONTANEOUS RECOVERY?

Reiki is not a miracle drug for all sorts of diseases, because Reiki is aimed at restoring the balance and this is often a long and slow process. This means that it needs time to "work." It has usually taken years to become unbalanced, so it will also take time and dedication to restore the balance.

Reiki can only support a process and is no replacement for regular medicine. The effects of Reiki on various types of minor ailments, such as aching muscles, headache, stomach/belly ache, tiredness and common cold (the so-called everyday ailments) are of course often immediately noticeable!

WHAT IS THE DIFFERENCE BETWEEN MAGNETIZING AND REIKI?

People who magnetize work with the same energy as people who use Reiki. However, if people who magnetize are not attuned properly to the energy field, it is possible that they give away their own energy supply. This has to do with the fact that they give away more than they are able to take in from the energy field. If you apply the Reiki method, you will never give away your own energy, because when giving a treatment, the energy will pass through your channel and therefore, you will receive (energy) at the same time. You will notice that, when you are tired and still decide to give someone else a treatment, you too will feel better after the treatment. That is not always the case with magnetizing, although there are undoubtedly examples of magnetizers who never suffer from energy loss, because they are by nature able to take in enough energy from the energy field.

MCS (MULTIPLE CHEMICAL SENSITIVITY)

People with Multiple Chemical Sensitivity become ill as soon as they are exposed to specific chemicals (smoke, perfume, cleaning products, et cetera). This is often caused by a problem in their detoxification system (sometimes caused by DNA defects) and/or for example short and long time chemical (over) exposure (think of the many firefighters who got ill after September 11 or of soldiers with Gulf War syndrome). Reiki cannot solve this problem, but it can support both the physical and mental processes and the energy deficiency that often occurs in this syndrome. A combination of remedies is best to try and improve the condition: avoid the chemical stimuli, eat biological food, use food supplements to support detoxification, exercise, meditate and use Reiki (see www.the-abc-of-mcs.com for more information about this disease).

273. Relationships

In any life relationships come and go, but unfortunately an MCS patient tends to see more going than coming. Almost every MCS patient has to face misunderstanding and the loss of contact with family and friends. It's important to above all never let your feeling of self-worth be affected by the departure of others and to become good company for yourself. You are worthy of having relationships; your illness just hampers them a little bit. When people leave you, view it as saying more about them than about yourself as a person. Not everyone is capable of associating with somebody with MCS. At all times, make sure you take good care of yourself; then at least you're guaranteed that amount of care. If you'd like to read more about loss and relationships, go to *Part II: The Personal Situation* and *Part III: The Voices of Others.*

274. Respiratory protection

There are various ways to protect your breathing and rid the air of the substances that are making you sick. You can use an MCS mask; a gassed-out gas mask (half or full face mask) with a filter screwed on; or a helmet with a motor-powered mobile air purifying system. When using protection involving loose filters it's best to choose the most all-encompassing filters so that a broad spectrum of chemical substances and gases is covered. Ask your supplier for advice.

No system covers everything. There are always substances which you react to that might not shielded by your filters, but in general these filters provide enough protection for MCS patients. If you know of any other substances which have to be purified from the air, discuss it extensively with a specialist in filter materials.

Below is an overview of the various possibilities:

MCS MASK

This is an example of an organic cotton mask with charcoal filling. For mild MCS patients this mask is often sufficient, but the more severe MCS patient usually needs heavier protection. It's best to choose an "official" MCS mask from MCS-specialized suppliers rather than a normal construction cotton mask from hardware stores because the materials will be safer. MCS masks are usually made without chemicals. You can buy MCS masks from these online sources: www.aehf.com, http://icanbreathe.com, www.needs.com.

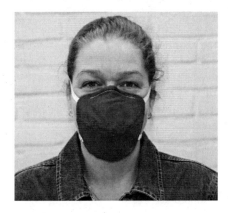

HALF/FULL FACE MASK

These masks can be found in hardware stores or online shops and are safe for use once they have been properly gassed out. They are not immediately safe because they are made using rubber, silicone and other synthetic substances. But, once they are out-gassed, all you have to do is screw on the filter and it's ready to go. Wearing these masks for a long time is not comfortable, so if it gets to the point where

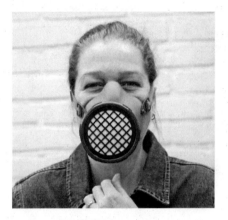

you're wearing it often and for long periods, you might want to choose the PAPR system, mentioned below.

Again: Consistently avoiding chemical substances will always be the safest and most effective approach!

Buy face masks for example from: www.msanorthamerica.com or www.lab safety.com/store/Safety_Supplies/Respirators/Air-Purifying_Respirators/?recs PerPage=45.

POWERED AIR PURIFYING RESPIRATOR (PAPR)

This system is a helmet connected to a mobile air purifier, which can be worn using a belt around the hips or in a backpack with enough holes for ventilation. It is attached to a flexible hose, which is snapped on at the back of the helmet. A constant supply of clean air emanates from the motor with the filter(s), through the hose and up to the helmet, creating a pressurized space that prevents outside gases from entering the helmet. This system provides good protection in emergency situations, on trips or in public places such as stores. Also see *entries 65 to 71* for more personal in-

formation about this system and experiences with its use.

The motor (mobile air purifier)

The motor with filter(s) can be used quickly after purchase without the hose. However, just to be safe, allow the engine to run and gas out in another room. The motor can be held on your lap, for example in the car or when making unsafe visits. The hip belt can be used for the motor, but the motor can also be worn in a backpack as long as it has enough holes for ventilation. In that case, use the flexible hose.

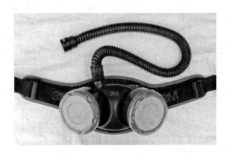

The helmet

The flexible hose takes a long time to gas out, sometimes up to a year, though this can be shortened by taking various measures or by using a somewhat sturdier hose. Heat helps air out the material. Place it outside in the sun or near other sources of heat. Do make sure that you won't be inhaling the gases that this releases. A warm bath (not too hot) with baking soda helps gas out the hose, and it can be hung outside under an awning for a long time without any problems.

If you are using the motor and the hose, but not the helmet, it might be a good idea to create some kind of necklace from a safe pliable material in which

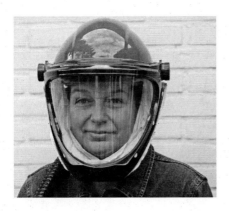

you can clasp the hose, so you can have two free hands while still maintaining a constant supply of purified air.

Some points of interest regarding the PAPR system:

• The system is not specifically designed for an MCS patient and it's therefore very important to completely gas the system out before taking it into use. Gassing out the hose can take up to a year.

• Wearing the system 24 hours a day is not advisable, so it's still important to make your own home 100 percent safe and to clean the air in your home using air purifiers.

• Not every MCS patient is ready to use or needs to use such a system; this not only depends on the severity of your MCS, but also on yourself, because you have to cross a high emotional hurdle in order to show yourself in public wearing a helmet. Usually this system is only used as a last recourse.

• Some people are very hesitant to use this system. Not everyone can tolerate the system very well, and the long-term consequences of its use are unknown. People worry that those who use the helmet might just become more sen-

sitive to synthetic and other substances. Yet some long-term users of the system have actually had very good experiences and they do not support this position. They feel the system has given them much more freedom. In summary, this product, just like every other product, has to be *fully* gassed out and should be used only if you are sure that you can tolerate it. In theory every product can be gassed out and made suitable for an MCS patient, including this one.

Following are links about masks and respirators.

POWERED AIR PURIFYING RESPIRATOR (PAPR)

www.3m.com
www.msanorthamerica.com/catalog/catalog526.html
www.westernsafety.com/3m/3mrespiratorypg4.html
www.safetycompany.com/powered-air-purifying-respirator-powered-air-purifying-respira/c_13_230_231.html?osCsid=801a7cbd01d5f1ae6c1a61ae3712169f

MASKS

www.respro.com
www.websoft-solutions.net/protective_respirators_safety_respirators_s/42.htm

Visit www.the-abc-of-mcs.com under "Breath" or see *Part VI: Further Resources* for more information on companies that sell MCS masks and other systems. If you'd like to exchange experiences on this subject with fellow patients, become a member of an online forum (see *entry 205*).

275. Sauna

The "Heavenly Heat" sauna is specially made for MCS patients out of white poplar wood, which does not make most MCS patients sick. It is a so-called "Finnish dry sauna" that is heated electrically, using stove with natural stones. The temperatures aren't as high as with a normal sauna, but that's actually better for an MCS patient and promotes detoxification. These sauna treatments can also be combined with Far Infrared therapy.

Also see *entry 182* about detoxification. Detoxification therapy (saunas, supplements, etc.) are best done under the supervision of an MCS specialist. There are a number of places where you can receive such supervision. Dr. Rea's book (see *entry 328*) offers a lot of information about the use of saunas for MCS patients. There is even a book specifically about saunas and their use: *Sauna Detoxification Therapy — A Guide for the Chemically Sensitive* by Marilyn McVicker (see *entry 333*).

For information on MCS saunas, visit www.the-abc-of-mcs.com under "Sauna," www.heavenlyheatsaunas.com, and www.greenlivingoasis.com/saunas.html.

276. Scent-free city

The only completely perfume-free and scent-free city is Halifax, Nova Scotia, although there are other cities discussing the issue, particularly Ottawa. The arguments in favor of making a city scent-free are, among others, that people have a right to breathe clean air and not be exposed to chemical scents that needlessly cause health problems. The chemicals in scented products can induce an asthma attack and other allergic reactions. To read more about the details with regard to Ottawa, visit www.ottawa.ca (search term: scent-free).

For various links to perfume-free initiatives, schools, churches, hospitals, and so on especially in the US and Canada, visit www.the-abc-of-mcs.com under "Perfume (free)" or see *Part VI*.

277. Scent marketing

More and more stores and companies are using scent devices or columns, to spread a certain smell in their shops or buildings, because this is supposed to have a stimulating impact on purchasing behavior (which confirms the argument that scents can influence our brain and behavior). These companies do not pause to consider that people with asthma and other respiratory problems can absolutely not tolerate these synthetic scents, and will get sick. These customers would actually rather avoid such stores. All we can do is write letters to prevent certain plans (such as in public spaces) from going through. Writing appears to work really well, especially when it can cost these companies clientele!

278. Schools

Some schools in the United States and Canada have gone perfume- and scent-free, but most still use plenty of perfumed cleaning products and air fresheners in the bathrooms and elsewhere. All you can do is write letters and send articles to the relevant schools about the consequences of chemical substances on the development of children.

Fortunately, there are plenty of examples of institutions that have become scent-free (see *entry 276*). It's all about raising consciousness. Try to inform many more parents, such that the school board can be convinced to make changes. Focus your activism on the health of the children, pointing to conditions such as asthma, allergies and respiratory problems. Put the emphasis on the use of chemicals, since those form a threat to everyone, not just MCS patients. See www.the-abc-of-mcs.com under "Perfume (free)" and *Part VI*. Get in touch with perfume-free schools in America and Canada and inquire about how they got it done and educated parents, teachers and students. They may have excellent informational materials to share with you.

279. Shoe polish

Olive oil and Vaseline are good substitutes for shoe polish. Be careful with Vaseline, though, it can cause a negative reaction, being made using petroleum. You can also find organic alternatives for shoe polish like the brand Tapir (see www.snappydressers.com). Other alternatives are to have your shoes polished by someone else (outside of the house) or to use good respiratory protection if you do it yourself. Do let your polished shoes gas out for a while before wearing them.

280. Shoes

New shoes should first be gassed out thoroughly, or you could choose shoes with less harmful materials, although this does not imply that they will be immediately suitable for an MCS patient. For example, the footbeds of Birkenstocks are made from recycled cork from the bottle industry, mixed with natural latex: www.birkenstockusa.com/green-steps. Shoes from Nike Considered are made of PVC-free leather, cotton and burlap. These shoes do not contain chemical glue substances and are tanned using vegetable oils. See http://store.nike.com.

For more information on several other brands, see: www.thegreenguide.com.

281. Shopping

Shopping unprotected is probably no longer doable, because in busy shopping streets you'll encounter quite a few perfume clouds and cigarette smoke. Some stores nowadays also spread scents in the air to entice customers, which can cause problems. If you can, shop online or ask someone else to go into town for you. There is a plethora of online options these days. See *Part VI* for several online stores.

282. Short-term memory

If you have a lot of problems with short-term memory, always carry with you a notepad and a pencil. Even if you consistently avoid chemicals this symptom might remain, since this can be the result of various exposures and isn't easily reversible.

Ultra Brain Power (American Biologics) is a supplement which (if you can tolerate it) might somewhat improve your memory. It's available at www.vitaminshoppe.com or www.needs.com.

283. Shortness of breath

Shortness of breath is often a consequence of exposure to chemical substances. Oxygen (see *entry 252*), can help relieve the problem, but it's always better to prevent exposure to irritants. See also www.the-abc-of-mcs.com under "Water & Oxygen."

284. Shower filter

In order to prevent a possible sensitive reaction to the chlorine in the water coming from the shower, you can have a chlorine filter installed on your shower. See these links: www.showerfilterstore.com; www.needs.com; www.healthgoods.com

285. Showering

When showering, use products that are suitable for you and do not let housemates use products that you can't tolerate. Also see *entry 284*.

286. Sinus infections

Sinus infections arise because chemical substances or allergens irritate the mucous membrane, causing an infection. For prevention or treatment, most people use a nasal spray with corticosteroids or other medicine. Clearly this would entail an added chemical burden for the MCS patient. Avoid them for as long as you can (consult your physician), but start looking for alternative substances that are just as effective. The best remedy for MCS patients is still just the consistent avoidance of irritating substances.

If you can tolerate tea tree oil (available at natural food stores), it's a good substance to use for preventing and curing infections (*not for internal use!!*). Rinse your nose and sinus cavities regularly with a few drops of tea tree oil added to a colloidal silver solution (about three drops per mug; this can be adjusted as you wish). In cases of sensitivity to tea tree oil, you can rinse with just the colloidal silver solution. Apply the solution using a syringe (without needle, of course) from the pharmacy. After stirring the solution, fill the syringe. Tilt your head to one side when squirting the solution up your nose, then bend over and hang your head upside down (as if you were intending to do a headstand). The solution will then also enter your frontal sinus cavity. Repeat process on the other side. This concoction does a great job of cleaning up infections and can also work to prevent them. Yet the emphasis should still be placed on avoiding all substances that cause infections.

Nasal irrigation with a saline solution helps as well.

If your nose or sinus cavities are swollen or irritated, the rinsing process can at first be quite painful, because of the added tea tree oil. This will get better over time and eventually even be painless, which is a good sign that things are getting back to normal. Choose an organic, 100 percent pure tea tree oil (see also *entry 19*).

In cases of nasal and sinus problems, often the Physiomer Gentle Jet Nasal Cleanser is used for rinsing. However, it is not recommended for use by MCS patients who react to rubber. Physiomer makes use of a "spherile system" instead of a gas propellant, meaning their bottle contains a rubber balloon that keeps the bottle under pressure until it is empty.

287. Smog

When temperatures rise in crowded industrial areas and cities and there is little wind, the result is an increase in the level of smog. You should not go outside on smoggy days, but instead stay inside as much as possible, with the windows and doors shut and the air purifiers running until it's over. Smog clears up automatically once the wind picks up or changes direction, or when it rains. Smog can cause brain fog (see *entry 162*), respiratory problems and other problems for MCS patients and certainly also for people who experience respiratory problems in general.

If you want to find what smog levels are and will be, see *Part VI* or the MCS website under "Air Pollution" for informative links.

288. Sodium bicarbonate

Also known as baking soda. See *entry 154*.

289. Sofa

A new sofa should be thoroughly gassed out for months in a room the MCS patient does not have to enter. When possible, choose sofas made using natural and chemical-free materials. This will shorten the gassing-out period or even make it unnecessary.

See also www.the-abc-of-mcs.com under "Living" or *Part VI*.

290. Spirituality

Listed below are a number of questions and answers taken (with permission) from the translated manuscript of *The ABCs of Reiki*.

WHAT IS SPIRITUALITY?

Spirituality means relating to the spirit, incorporeal. Spirituality is therefore not matter, it is not about material things and you cannot really put your finger on it. It is something that takes place in the mind. Spirituality has a different meaning, a different feel for everyone, although we are all talking about the same essence using different words.

WHAT IS THE POINT OF SPIRITUAL DEVELOPMENT?

In my view, spirituality is the way inside and a way to become a happier person by working on yourself and becoming aware of who you are. By working on your awareness processes you change and this way you have a huge effect on your environment. "Change the world, start with yourself" thus gets a deep meaning.

DOES REIKI DEVELOP YOUR SPIRITUALITY?

Reiki is a way to develop your spiritual awareness.

A lot of people find that Reiki is a method to get more in touch with themselves. This is also described as returning to your feelings or your Inner Self. The more in touch you get with your feelings, the more intuitive and the more aware you become.

Awareness is the ability to be conscious. Awareness is the first step to (spiritual) development, also called change or transformation. Spiritual development has a different dimension for everyone. Some people will look for God in church and some people will find God (or the source) in the silence within, independent of all religions.

HOW DO YOU DEVELOP YOUR SPIRITUALITY?

• By treating yourself with energy on a regular basis you get more in touch with yourself, which in turn has an effect on your spiritual awareness.

• Meditating, like Reiki, promotes spiritual growth.

• Prayer is another way to breathe new life into your spirituality.

• Thankfulness and submission are two aspects that support your spiritual awareness. We hardly ever ask ourselves why we are here and what our tasks are. How special it is to be a part of the great mystery called life. Being thankful for all the experiences of life will bring you spiritual depth. After all, your experiences have formed you, have taught you something and have brought you here.

• Counting your blessings every day is another beautiful way to live your life with more awareness and thus strengthen your spirituality.

291. Stoves

Thoroughly protect yourself against the (stove) smoke in your surroundings by sealing your house and by using good air purifiers. In general, complaining to your neighbors won't be of much use: in the winter people will want to stoke their wood stoves or fireplaces and in the summer they'll want to barbecue or light their fire pits. If you're lucky, you'll have neighbors who are well informed of your health and are willing to be considerate of you. Often it makes a big difference if your neighbors are willing to warn you when they plan to light a fire. Yet most people won't take you seriously right away. They also might feel that you are limiting their freedom, a sentiment that can easily sour neighborly relations. You should only consider moving to an other home if it will be a move to a relatively quiet place where neighbors are scarce. However, even this is not a guarantee that the air is clean in the wintertime and that your home won't be polluted.

292. Stress

Stress can worsen your MCS-related ailments due to the adrenaline boosts (internal irritants) which your body has to process. Especially in case of a damaged detoxification system, this can mean an added burden. Meditation and Reiki are quick methods for relaxing a body and mind that is stressed (see entries *238* and *272*).

293. Sugar

In order not to burden your body with chemical substances, it's advisable to always choose organic sugars. There are lots of options at natural foods stores. Refined sugars have undergone a chemical process and should be avoided. Some examples of refined sugars are white sugar (crystal sugar), grape sugar, dextrose, glucose and sweeteners such as maltitol and sorbitol. Natural sugars tend not to be bad for you; they're found in grains, fruits and sweet vegetables. Healthy alternatives are raw sugars, fruit juice concentrate, maple syrup and honey. Ask for advice in a natural foods store or from the environmental health therapist or doctor.

294. Sweeteners

See *entry 293.*

295. Synthetic materials

Try to avoid new synthetic materials as much as possible, or always let them thoroughly gas out before taking them into use. In theory, all materials can be gassed out. How long this process takes depends on the product. Generally speaking, hard materials are safe for use sooner than softer synthetic materials.

296. Tampons and menstrual pads

NatraCare tampons and menstrual pads are entirely made of organic and natural materials. The brand is available in natural stores and also online, at www.alyahs.com, for example. Visit www.natracare.com for more information on the products themselves. You can also purchase washable organic cotton menstrual pads at www.hankettes.com and http://manymoonsalternatives.com. Also see *entry 371.*

297. Tea tree oil

Long before Captain Cook discovered Australia and drank tea made from the leaves of the tea tree, Australian Aboriginals used the leaves of this tree for various purposes, including its healing properties. The leaves were ground up and formed into packages with clay, which were used to treat all kinds of skin conditions and infections. Tea tree oil is suited for very many purposes. In diluted form it can be used to rinse cavities, and in either its pure or diluted form it can be applied to skin to treat rashes and itches. Tea tree oil has disinfecting effects, kills mold and has countless other possible applications. Several books about the many possible uses of tea tree oil are available. For examples, search for "tea tree oil" online. If you are able to tolerate tea tree oil, always choose a pure and organic brand.

298. Tests

Most homeopathic and orthomolecular doctors, therapists and clinics, will test you for, among other things, shortages and excesses of vitamins, minerals, and amino acids. This can be very useful, assuming the doctor or therapist in question has an understanding of MCS. Yet in practice, many costly tests deliver poor results because the MCS patient experiences problems with the prescribed food supplements. These supplements may give you a poisoning or intolerance reaction. It's advisable to approach everything with restraint and, above all, slowly build up the dosage. Below are a few options where you can find treatment from doctors who have knowledge of environmental sensitivities.

ENVIRONMENTAL
HEALTH CENTERS

Make sure you research them thoroughly with questions about how they can help before you make your final decision to become a patient.

Environmental Health Center
   Dallas, TX
   William J. Rea, M.D.
   www.ehcd.com
   Phone: (214) 368-4132

Center for Occupational & Environmental Medicine
   North Charleston, SC
   Allan D. Lieberman, M.D.
   http://coem.com
   Phone: (843) 572-1600

The Nova Scotia Environmental Health Centre
   Fall River, NS, Canada
   www.cdha.nshealth.ca
   Phone: (902) 860-0057

The Environmental Health Center at the Woman's College Hospital
   Toronto, ON
   www.womenshealthmatters.ca/Centres/environmental
   Phone: (416) 351-3764

Breakspear Hospital
   England
   Dr. Jean Monro
   www.breakspearmedical.com
   Phone: +44-1442-261-333

Also see *question 15* for more environmental health centers.

SOME WELL-KNOWN DOCTORS, PHYSICIANS AND THERAPISTS

Doris J. Rapp, M.D.
   www.drrapp.com

Gunnar Heuser, M.D., Ph.D., F.A.C.P.
   www.toxgun.com

ORGANIZATIONS

Environmental Medicine Physicians
   http://mcs-america.org/doctorlist.pdf

American Academy of Environmental Medicine
   Wichita, KS
   www.aaemonline.org
   Phone: (316) 684-5500

Association of Occupational and Environmental Clinics
   Washington, DC
   www.aoec.org
   Phone: (202) 347-4976

For laboratories see *Part VI*.

299. Therapies and Therapists

When you are looking for a therapy or therapist, the best advice is to go to an environmental health specialist to get your MCS diagnosed and to get the proper treatment. Some patients pursue other therapies in search of improvement. You can follow many therapies and visit many therapists, all of whom could possibly bring about improvement to your situation. Although MCS is a chronic condition (see *entry 24*), certain therapies can be very effective in treating specific symptoms and ailments. The most important thing to keep in mind is that what worked well for someone else does not necessarily have to work for you (or can even be counterproductive). No two MCS patients are alike; MCS is a multiple-system disease, meaning all organs can be involved in this clinical picture, resulting in an enormous variety of symptoms.

Above all, remember that at a certain point it becomes best to focus your energy toward finding betterment (with or without the help of therapy) and toward adjusting your life. Also very important is acceptance, which brings inner peace, which in turn is good for your general wellbeing. Also see *entry 21* with regard to which therapies are considered useful by MCS patients (research among almost 1,000 patients).

One warning should be issued. Before adopting any therapy, you should be careful to first get information and inquire among other patients as to their experiences. Even though everyone is unique, useful information can still come to light. It's important to calmly acquire information and make sure that the practice of the doctor or therapist who you'll be visiting regularly is somewhat adjusted to your needs, or visit while wearing protection. It would be a shame if these outings were to saddle you with all sorts of irritants instead of improvement.

300. Toilet paper

Use chlorine-free, perfume-free recycled toilet paper (available in natural stores and in some supermarkets) in order to spare the skin.

301. Traveling

If you have MCS it's definitely no longer easy to travel by airplane, assuming you're even still capable of leaving the house. Airplane cabins can, among other things, be sprayed with pesticides and on top of that, you're in a small, poorly ventilated space close to other people and their perfumes and other chemical substances. The air is not rich in oxygen, and the materials in the cabin contain many brominated flame retardants, both of which can cause problems. Even flight attendants and pilots can become ill because of frequent airplane travel. Nevertheless, there are various ways to fly without experiencing too many negative consequences. These measures are of course strongly dependent on the severity of the developed MCS, although they could also be seen as a way to prevent deterioration.

• First of all, protect yourself by wearing a respirator mask or a helmet with a mobile air purifier or, if you're a "mild" MCS patient, by wearing a cotton MCS mask. (See *entry 274.*) You may wish to bring a doctor's letter explaining you must wear the respirator for medical reasons.
• Make sure that your skin is covered as much as possible by, for example, wearing Tyvek coveralls. (See *entry 306.*)
• Cover your hair with a scarf or hat.
• You might be able to arrange extra oxygen on board (request it beforehand and make sure you have a letter from your doctor). Bring your own ceramic oxygen mask and possibly a Tygon tube. Bringing your own oxygen tends to be forbidden, although the FAA-approved (Federal Aviation Administration) oxygen concentrator is usually allowed. For more information, see: www.continental.com/web/en-US/content/travel/specialneeds/disabilities/customer_oxygen.aspx. Research this problem thoroughly beforehand with the airline you plan to fly! See *entry 252* about oxygen.

• Bring tri-salts (see *entry 302*) in order to quickly neutralize any possible negative reactions.

• Bring your own soap and towels and wash your face and uncovered skin repeatedly throughout the journey.

• Bring your own lunch or other edibles rather than consuming the airplane food. Do inquire beforehand whether or not this is permitted on your flight, since many countries do not allow food items to be imported. But usually you can eat any items brought on board during the flight.

• You can ask the flight attendants beforehand if you can sit in the very front (get on the plane last) and disembark first in order to avoid getting entangled in a mass of people.

• If the plane is not fully booked, try to ensure that you have no one sitting next to you. Arrange it with the flight crew beforehand that if someone wearing perfume sits next to you, the crew will find a different seat either for you or for that person.

• As soon as you arrive, wash your hair and skin in order to rinse off the harmful substances as soon as possible. Immediately changing your clothes is also advisable.

• If, upon arrival, you've arranged for a rental car, make sure you tell the rental agency to reserve you an old car in which nothing is sprayed, cleaning detergents have not recently been applied and there is no air freshener.

Here are a few links about air travel (also see *entry 378*): www.flyana.com; www.flying-with-disability.org; http://mcstravel.resourcez.com.

TIPS

• It's safest to travel in your own gassed-out safe car, a gassed-out trailer or your own tailor-made RV. While on the road, it's a good idea to push the air-conditioning "recycle" button while in busy areas, so no exhaust fumes enter inside. Using a mobile air purifier is really a must. Also see *entry 168*.

• Using public toilets is not a good idea for MCS patients because of the chemicals (perfume, air fresheners, cleaning detergents, etc.) which users will encounter. Urinating outside or using a urine spout (for women) is an excellent solution to this problem. See www.pmateusa.com for more information. There are also possibilities for in the car, such as the Uribag F urine bag for women, available at drug stores or http://elderstore.com/uribag-female.aspx.

• See also *entry 217* about hotels.

302. Tri-salts

In order to neutralize a negative physical reaction, you can use tri-salts. This is a combination of calcium (carbonate), magnesium (carbonate) and potassium (bicarbonate). Tri-salts lower the acid content in the body so that chemical substances can be removed more effectively and the physical reaction to chemical substances will thus not last as long.

The acid/alkaline content can be checked using pH sticks, which measure the content levels in the urine (these sticks can be ordered at the pharmacy). The normal pH level lies between 6.5 and 8.5. An MCS patient often displays a level that is too acidic, sometimes even below 5.0. Dr. Rea advises the use of tri-salts to his patients (see *entry 328*). Tri-salts are available at the pharmacy or at several online stores (see links below).

INSTRUCTIONS FOR USE
(OR FOLLOW THE ADVICE OF
YOUR THERAPIST/DOCTOR):

Tri-salts for daily use: half a teaspoon dissolved into a glass of water. Start with one-third or one-quarter teaspoon and gradually build up the dose.

Tri-salts for acute reactions: take the highest dose that you can tolerate in one go. Too high a dose leads to diarrhea! If the reaction does not recede, repeat this process after two hours, up to five times in ten hours.

Tri-salts for use with sauna therapy: in all cases take tri-salts beforehand and, in case of a reaction, also after being in the sauna.

The brand Ecological Formulas (tri-salts 200 grams) does not contain the composite sodium bicarbonate (baking soda). If you use tri-salts products or recipes that include baking soda, discuss them with a doctor in case of kidney problems and heart diseases or high blood pressure.

The frequent use of tri-salts as well as the process of detoxification depletes more vitamins than usual, thus it's advisable to take extra vitamins. Ask your therapist or doctor for advice.

LINKS

Ph Sticks:

http://healthyover50.net/phsticks.htm

Tri-salts:

www.needs.com/product/Ecologi cal_Formulas_Tri_Salts_200/vspgb_Eco logical_Formulas

http://store.agoodvitamin.com/ec fotr200mg.html

www.absolutelythepurest.com/supp lements/Tri%20Salts.html

303. TV

See *entry 191*.

304. TV Guide

See *entry 221*.

305. Tygon tube

MCS patients use this type of tube to connect the oxygen tank (see *entry 252*) to the mask (see *entry 171*). This tube is available from the American Environmental Health Foundation, founded by Dr. Rea. For more information, see www.aehf.com/catalog/product_info. php?products_id=916.

306. Tyvek

Tyvek is a material (polyethylene or PE) to which MCS patient usually respond well. It is effective in protecting yourself or your safe furniture from chemical substances (such as your couch or chair in times of "unsafe" visitors). The product is scentless. The smooth side does not allow gases to pass through, allowing it to become the "unsafe" contact side. Tyvek is available from kite-making and repair shops. For example, see: www.intothewind.com/ shop/Repair_and_Kitemaking/Fabric/T yvek. Tyvek coveralls are available from,

among other places, www.abcsafety
mart.com/clothing/clothing.html and
www.tasco-safety.com/tyvek-protective-
clothing.html.

307. Vacation

Going on vacation is not simple and
can be downright impossible if you're a
severe MCS patient. If you're somebody
who can still leave home, then there are
some options as to ecological vacation
resorts. Non-ecological lodgings are not
recommended, because you'll then have
to deal with vacation homes or hotel
rooms that are cleaned with synthetic
products. The bedding will usually have
been washed using common (synthetic)
laundry detergents, but actually bedding
is the easiest thing to deal with, because
you can bring your own. Of course,
avoid anyplace where smoking is
permitted. When you think you've
found a place you can stay, it's a good
idea to ask questions beforehand on
what the situation is at the given establishment and to thoroughly explain your
condition.

LINKS

www.safertraveldirectory.com
www.thenaturalplace.com
http://health.groups.yahoo.com/grou
p/mcssafeshelterusa/
http://yellowcanary.com/travelsafe/

Also see *entry 301* for tips on travel by
airplane or car/RV and *Part VI*.

308. Ventilation

It's very important to keep ventilat-
ing, among other things to keep mold
from growing in your home. Try to
open your doors and windows as much
and often as possible during "safe"
hours.

309. Vermin and pests

See *entry 263*.

310. Visitors

If you'd like to receive guests without
experiencing harmful consequences, it's
best to give your guests a list of instructions beforehand (after finding out to
what extent your guest is willing to
make adjustments). It's up to you to decide how high to set the bar, but do realize that after each new exposure you
could become more sensitive to even
more substances. Eventually the price
may become too steep (being sick for a
few days or even a week as a result of
one visit from someone who wore perfume or aftershave). By guarding your
own boundaries like a watchdog, you
learn to stand up for yourself and you
create a safer life for yourself, which has
positive effects upon your general well-
being. See *entry 225* for a list of instructions.

If you have contractors or repairmen
come over, you can very easily make an
agreement with the company that their
employees not wear aftershave or smoke
right before arriving. You should, of
course, keep protecting yourself during
their visit, because their clothes and

such have not been adjusted. But at least you will have prevented pure perfume or fumes from cigarette smoke from being brought into your home. Or, if a contractor has to come to your house often, you can give him the products you use so that he can wash his clothes and himself with them. This reduces a large part of the burden. And often they're willing to cooperate, especially when it doesn't cost them a thing. Another option with regard to their clothing is to have them pull on Tyvek coveralls (see *entry 306*).

311. Walls

Products for covering walls such as wallpaper and paint contain chemical substances and are therefore best avoided, as with their use you run the risk of no longer being able to spend time in that particular room. Synthetic wallpaper is often treated with mold-preventing products. The heavier the wallpaper, the more chemical substances are in the glue in order to keep it on the wall. It's therefore best to choose natural paint or a purely natural product, such as natural plaster, caulk or loam. Even with natural products, it's still a good idea to first test them thoroughly by putting some on a piece of safe wood, to see if you can tolerate it (by putting the piece of wood beside your bed, for example).

Visit www.the-abc-of-mcs.com under "Living" or see *Part VI* for various websites which can inform you on this subject. Keep in mind that "green" does not imply the product is nontoxic or suitable for MCS patients. Be careful with everything you want to change in the house, especially when renovating.

312. Water purification

Filter your water by means of a water purification system or drink only mineral water in glass bottles. Tap water is purified using chemical substances including chlorine, that may be within the allowable limits but can still be taxing to MCS patients.

When buying a purification system, choose a good steel, ceramic and charcoal water system. For examples or more information, go to: www.aehf.com (see water filters), www.needs.com (see water purifiers), www.purewaterplace.com, or www.cleanairpurewater.com.

313. Workplace

If you still work outside the home, you have no choice but to bring your superiors and colleagues up to speed on MCS. Try to foster sympathy for your situation and educate them about MCS, though this won't always be easy, depending on the attitude of the people you work with. Perhaps a move to a separate space would be possible, in which you could place a portable air purifier. You could also ask your colleagues not to enter your office if they're wearing perfume and request that they primarily use the phone to contact you. Don't forget to put a sign on your door and perhaps protect yourself with a mask or a helmet when walking through the building. In many situations an MCS patient will have to look for a different workplace where your sensitivities won't be as much of a problem. There aren't very many of these, so working at home is one of the best options. There are ways to adjust your current workplace; visit this informative link: Canadian Human Rights Commission, www.chrcccdp.ca/pdf/envsensitivity_en.pdf.

314. Yeast infections

See *entry 166.*

PART V
Films, Books and Other Resources

14

Films

315. Canary in the Mine

www.afc.gov.au/filmsandawards/filmdb
search.aspx?view=title&title=CANAIN
1997, VHS PAL (Australia)

This is a very moving film about a 17-year-old boy in isolation. He can only receive guests while wearing a helmet with an air purification system. Ever since childhood he has had to wear an air purification device on his back. At home, he makes use of various air purification devices and always carries around a hose which supplies purified air. He has not been outside in more than eight years. He has DNA deficiencies and his father worked with chemical substances, which according to the movie accounts for this boy's disorders.

I was able to relate very strongly to this movie, among other things due to the use of the helmet. My grandfather was a painter and thus worked with many solvents and other chemical substances. This may have produced genetic changes in his children. The movie made me realize once more that MCS is a slow, steady, inevitable process.

Conclusion: good film
Language: English

316. Chemical Injury Conference, October 2003, in Fairfax, Virginia

This almost-17-hour long conference is available on DVD and videotape. This conference brought together many experts (Meggs, Ziem, Kilburn, Rea, Morton, Pall, Baker, the Andersons and many more) to discuss MCS and related conditions. It contains a great deal of interesting information. The Chemical Injury Information Network (CIIN) sells the tapes and DVDs, but the quality of the recordings is not quite what it should be. The recordings were made from the back of the room, so a lot of the audio and video quality was lost, making some sections hard to follow.

Conclusion: good conference, poor sound quality
Language: English

317. Chemical Kids

This is a Danish documentary from 2001 about the dangers of chemical substances in our environment and the impact that they have on us and our (unborn) children. This documentary must certainly have been an eye opener for many people and must have led to changes in people's behavior.

Helle Kongevang (see *entry 102*) makes an appearance, as do various experts in the field of the environment, politics, chemistry and science.

The following links offer more information on the documentary: www.mediarights.org/film/chemical_kids and www.filmakers.com/index.php?a=film Detail&filmID=1053.

Conclusion: very good documentary
Languages: English and Danish

318. *Exposed*

www.exposed.at

Exposed is a beautiful movie (40 minutes long) about an American MCS patient. The protagonist, a professional dancer, often filmed herself throughout her life. She kept doing so when she developed MCS, and thereby documented on tape very intense emotions, thoughts out loud, and so on. Some moments were very moving and touched me deeply. The filmmaker intersperses the patient's own recordings with old commercials about chemicals, interviews, and other material.

This movie is definitely recommended for everyone. It can be ordered from the filmmaker, Heidrun Holzfeind, who can be reached through the website www.exposed.at.

Conclusion: good film
Language: English

319. *Final Insult*

www.roninfilms.com.au/video/1871977/0/1832141.html
1997, VHS PAL (Australia)

This is a very good Australian film about MCS and the environmental consequences of countless untested, potentially toxic chemical substances circulating in our surroundings every day. We are involved in a massive and dangerous experiment. How can we know for sure that our bodies can handle all this? The story about the canaries in the mine also features in this movie.

This is a multifaceted, moving film, giving voice to patients, doctors and experts (including Dr. Rea). It also follows a man as he is tested in clinic similar to Dr. Rea's. The movie shows his reactions to chemical substances.

Conclusion: very good film
Language: English

320. *Funny, You Don't Look Sick*

www.susanabod.com/funny.html

This film is the personal account of Susan Abod, an MCS/CFS patient, over a period of 18 months. Susan invites the viewer into her home and her life. In the movie, Susan discusses her life, the adjustments she has had to make, and her limitations. We're also taken along to her therapist and to a support group of which she is a member. The film can be ordered from Susan Abod herself.

Conclusion: good film
Language: English

321. *MCS: How Chemical Exposures May Be Affecting Your Health*

www.alisonjohnsonmcs.com

An excellent and very informative documentary about MCS, which is especially useful as an introduction for those who have just discovered MCS. You hear from many MCS patients as well as six leading medical experts in the field of MCS. If you are newly diagnosed, hearing others' stories will provide some degree of consolation. You are not alone. The DVD is available online through the website mentioned above.

Conclusion: excellent documentary
Language: English

322. [SAFE]

www.sonypictures.com/classics/safe/safe
.html

The movie [SAFE], starring Julianne Moore, actually starts off well (recognizable moments, the loneliness and lack of sympathy inherent to MCS), but it ends oddly involving some kind of spiritual therapy in New Mexico. The filmmaker appears to let his own conviction surface through the therapist — that you are the cause of your own illness and that it's all because you don't love yourself enough. That was a real turnoff (although some MCS patients fall into the hands of such "therapists" who convince them of all sorts of things).

The movie had a lot more potential, and could have projected a better message. It might have been improved with some useful information, but it is after all a feature film and not a documentary. [SAFE] is available at movie rental stores and various stores that sell movies.

Conclusion: somewhat relevant, but overall a very strange film
Language: English

323. *The Tomato Effect*

A shocking documentary about the suspicious death of Zane R. Kime, M.D. His daughter Faun Kime undertook a search for the cause of his death.

Did he fall from a mountain or was he pushed, and thus murdered?

Zane Kime was a doctor who concerned himself with MCS, treating patients and making diagnoses. He was a member of the AAEM (see *question 15*). At the time of his death he was wrapped up in the middle of lawsuit.

This film is about this quest for truth and about the many doctors who lost their licenses for having concerned themselves with environmental medicine and chemical illness — and who continue to do so. The film discusses the backlashes and lawsuits, the MCS patients, the reasons why MCS is still not recognized despite the existence of very thorough reports and evidence, the provocation test, and so on. www.satori-5.co.uk/word_articles/mcs/tomato_ef fect.html; www.mcs-international.org/vv_alternative_health/the_tomato_eff ect_trailer.html

324. *The Toxic Clouds of 9/11: A Looming Health Disaster*

www.alisonjohnsonmcs.com

The documentary opens with a steelworker who volunteered many hours to help clean up the wreckage of the 9/11 attacks. These cleanup activities after the disaster have had severe consequences for the rescue workers, surrounding residents, firemen, steelworkers, salvage workers, and others. Official health agencies declared the air safe without grounding their ruling in solid research or test results. As a result, few people wore protective masks while working. Furthermore, the people living near Ground Zero had to clean the chemical dust from their homes themselves.

The consequences cannot yet be comprehended and will keep affecting lives for decades to come, especially because there are still many toxic substances in the ventilation systems of the buildings in Manhattan. Nothing at all has been done about this. MCS comes into view halfway through the movie, because all these people have developed severe health problems and sensitivities to chemical substances. Their lives are forever marked, and a number of people have died as a result of being exposed to these chemical substances.

This is a shocking documentary, of course due to the disaster itself but also its horrible consequences. These celebrated heroes still receive no help from any institution whatsoever and are being completely left to their fate. Many have lost their health or their income or, because of their problems, are earning just a fraction of what they once did. Aside from all these things, this documentary is also relevant to many MCS patients due to the personal stories and the health problems it portrays.

This excellent film will endow viewers with greater understanding of the fact that chemical substances can make you sick.

Conclusion: very good documentary
Language: English

15

A Few Books About MCS

I have read and recommend the following nine books.

325. *Allergic to the Twentieth Century*
Peter Radetsky
Little Brown & Co.
264 pages

This book is about subjects including sick building syndrome, Gulf War syndrome and MCS and is filled with patients' stories, conversations with doctors, scientists, and skeptics. It is very readable (not a textbook). Available on Amazon.com and elsewhere.

326. *Casualties of Progress: Personal Histories from the Chemically Sensitive*
Alison Johnson, B.A., M.A.
MCS Information Exchange
276 pages

This book contains 57 stories of MCS patients from different backgrounds, such as doctors, industrial workers, nurses, painters, computer engineers, teachers, professors, psychologists, stock traders, students, lawyers, and Gulf War veterans. Even a few children voice their experiences.

Reading the stories of other MCS patients can at least provide a certain amount of consolation. The recognition and validation that are hard to find in daily life can often be found in the stories of others.

Sixteen of these patients also feature in the documentary MCS: How Chemical Exposures May Be Affecting Your Health (see *entry 321.*) Available on Amazon.com and on www.alisonjohnsonmcs.com.

327. *Chemical Exposures: Low levels and High Stakes*
Claudia S. Miller, M.D., M.S., and Nicholas A. Ashford, Ph.D., J.D.
Wiley Interscience
464 pages

A very good book which clarifies a great number of things, especially the acknowledgement and recognition of MCS, which is comforting for those who have just discovered it. It is scientifically written but is still accessible to the lay person. Absolutely recommended for doctors and therapists as well. Available on Amazon.com and elsewhere.

328. *Chemical Sensitivity: Tools for Diagnosis and Methods of Treatment, Volume IV*
William J. Rea, M.D.
CRC Press
928 pages

A must-have for all MCS patients, therapists and doctors. This scientific book contains everything about the diagnosis and the treatment of MCS. This book holds information about studies on more than twenty thousand MCS patients in the EHC in Dallas, summarizes lab tests, sauna detoxification therapy, exercises, lists of construction materials both dangerous and safe for MCS patients, the food supplements used, and so on. This is the last volume in a four-book series. Available on Amazon.com and on www.aehf.com (clinic in Dallas).

329. *Comfort in the Storm: Devotions for the Chemically Sensitive*

Janine Ridings
Pleasant Word
308 pages

The writer, an MCS patient, uses Bible citations and other quotations related to the situation of an MCS patient. The stories can be very helpful for those with spiritual or Christian religious convictions. For those who seek strength in their faith or spirituality, this book is definitely recommended. For more information: www.aromaofchrist.com/comfort_in_the_storm.htm. Available on www.amazon.com and also available as an E-book.

330. *Detoxify or Die*

Sherry A. Rogers, M.D.
Prestige Publications
409 pages

As the title suggests, this book emphasizes the importance of detoxification. First, the author recounts how the toxic substances which we store in our bodies (sometimes permanently), are pervasive everywhere in the world. The author talks about phases I and II of detoxification and about how toxic substances are the most important cause of most diseases. In conclusion, she offers instructions on how best to detoxify, such as with the aid of a sauna. Various sauna therapies and accompanying supplements are discussed. Available on Amazon.com and elsewhere.

(This author also wrote a small booklet entitled: "Chemical Sensitivity, Environmental Diseases and Pollutants: How They Hurt Us, How to Deal with Them." Just 47 pages long, it is a good resource for those who do not want to put the time and effort into something more thorough, but want to be well informed.)

331. *Free to Fly: A Journey toward Wellness*

Judit Rajhathy
New World Publishing
352 pages

A novel about one MCS patient's search for improvement for herself and her children, who fell ill from exposure to pesticides. The reader is taken along on her visits to all kinds of doctors and alternative therapists. The book extensively chronicles both her positive and negative experiences, and it is sprinkled with useful tips and advice. Available on Amazon.com and elsewhere.

332. *Our Toxic World: A Wake-Up Call*

Doris J. Rapp, M.D.
Environmental Research Foundation
511 pages

I have met Doris Rapp in person and I find her a fantastic woman. She's an incredibly kind and courageous woman. She is very committed and passionate, and one of her most important goals is raising consciousness about the (potential) dangers in the use of chemical substances all over the world. She writes about and for MCS patients and how chemical substances harm all of us (the wake up call!). She also writes about the evidence of substances found in wild animals and their consequences for these animals; the genetic changes in humans and animals as a result of chemical substances; about chemical substances themselves, lab results, and many studies and evidence. She also gives tips for living a life without harmful chemicals. This book is definitely a must-read! Available on amazon.com or on Doris Rapp's home page: www.drrapp.com/ourtoxicworld.htm.

333. *Sauna Detoxification Therapy: A Guide for the Chemically Sensitive*

Marilyn McVicker
McFarland
175 pages

This book is specifically written for MCS patients who want to start detox-

ifying with the aid of a sauna. The book first explains what MCS is, then talks about the dangers of chemicals and about the studies that have been conducted into the effects of detoxification for MCS patients. The detoxification process is clarified and various kinds of saunas and different therapy programs are discussed. A large portion of the book is also about building your own sauna. Available on Amazon.com or at www.mcfarlandpub.com.

The following is an overview of a number of other well-known books on MCS (which I have not yet read).

An Alternative Approach to Allergies
Theron G. Randolph, M.D., and Ralph W. Moss, Ph.D.

Canary in the Courtroom
Jessie MacLeod

Explaining Unexplained Illnesses: Disease Paradigm for Chronic Fatigue Syndrome, Multiple Chemical Sensitivity
Martin L. Pall (see *question 27*)

Multiple Chemical Sensitivity: A Survival Guide
Pamela Reed Gibson, Ph.D.

Staying Well in a Toxic World
Lynn Lawson

For more book suggestions, go to www.geocities.com/mcsworld2000/books_to_check_out.htm and www.mcs-global.org/Books_Publications.htm.

16

Art and Music

334. Kim Palmer, 1954–2006, USA

Kim Palmer was living in an RV in a small plot on the Arizona desert, completely exiled due to her MCS, when in 2006, at the age of 52, she passed away when her body finally gave up. During the last two years of her life she had also become electro-sensitive, which even further limited her life. (Also see *entry 128*.)

Her CD *Songs from a Porcelain Trailer* is specifically about MCS and about life in isolation, although her other CDs also contain many wonderful songs. As an MCS patient you'll find a great deal of recognition and consolation in these songs! Her pieces can move you to tears (see *question 86*). If you'd like to know more about this beautiful MCS-inspired music, go to www.kimpalmersongs.com. On this site you can download songs from two of her albums.

For lyrics from *Songs from a Porcelain Trailer*, go to www.citlink.net/~bhima/kim.htm

335. Mirjam Ruijter, the Netherlands

Gone Bananas? Gone Bananas!
http://mirjam-gone-bananas-english.blogspot.com/

Mirjam started this project during her stay among the banana plantations of Thailand, where she fled to as a result of having MCS. There she made beautiful artistic photos of the banana plantations, which she now uses to make her postcards. It's surprising how much beauty can reside in just one plant. She produces these postcards using a special printer that prints in three layers of color and finishes the pictures with a protective layering, resulting in a very durable product.

The back of the cards contain information about MCS including web links. You can use the postcards to inform recipients about MCS, partially thanks to the online links included on the card. Profits from the sales of "Gone Bananas" help Mirjam cover the costs of her travel, as she attends meetings worldwide to raise the public profile of MCS and increase consciousness, hoping to achieve full recognition for this condition very soon!

Read more of her story at *entry 117*.

336. Moon McNeill, Germany

Moon is an artist, MCS patient and founder of Creative Canaries, an organization for artists with MCS. Moon herself makes fantastic paintings, photographs, MCS posters, and T-shirts. Visit www.moonmcneill.de and www.creativecanaries.org for more information about her, her work, and her organization. Also see *entry 103* with regard to her life story.

337. Treesha deFrance, USA

Treesha is also a very creative canary. Her health was normal until she attended art school at the age of 38. There she started getting headaches and struggled with fatigue, which eventually was so bad she was forced to stay in bed due to persistent severe dizziness and frailty. For a year and a half she dragged herself from doctor to doctor in vain, before finally consulting a holistic doctor, who did testing to get at the root of the problem. She explained to Treesha how toxic the classroom must have been from the use of various chemical substances in the art supplies. Treesha received advice as to how she could regain her health, for example by eating organic food and consistently avoiding chemical substances in cleaning detergents, care products, clothing, furniture, and construction materials. Treesha's health never really recovered, but her situation did improve quite a bit. Treesha is now a musician, producer and an award-winning MCS cartoonist (see her websites for more information): http://treesha6.tripod.com; http://myspace.com/mcscomics; http://myspace.com/treeshasmusic; www.citlink.net/~bhima/treesha.htm.

338. Creative Canaries

www.creativecanaries.org

This network of artists with MCS was founded by Moon McNeill (see *entry 336*), and is intended to allow MCS artists to meet each other online. In this way they find similar people and discover ways to sell their artwork, exchange knowledge regarding safe materials, and so on. Together, they aim to earn recognition for MCS through their art, music and other talents such as writing. One forum for creative canaries is at http://health.groups.yahoo.com/group/CreativeCanariesCommunity.

More links and information on the many creative canaries: Various artists and their work: www.citlink.net/~bhima/artists.htm; An organization where you too can let your creativity run free: www.planetthrive.com; Humor and MCS (Sharon Wachsler): www.sickhumorpostcards.com; Links related to MCS t-shirts, etc.: www.cafepress.com/buy/canary/multiple+chemical+sensitivity; www.cafepress.com/zonas_mcs; Link to E-cards for MCS patients: http://toxicamenders.googlepages.com/toxicamenderse-greetingcards

17

Spiritual Nourishment

339. Mental Exercises

Emotions are derived from thoughts. There is always first a thought followed by an emotion. Being able to control your thoughts will allow you to determine a large portion of your sense of happiness. When you exchange a negative thought pattern for a positive one, you'll immediately notice the effects this has on your disposition. Thought patterns are stubborn, but can certainly be changed.

You can train yourself in this. Whenever you hear yourself make a negative statement, interrupt yourself right away, even if it's in the middle of a sentence. More and more you'll realize you can indeed exercise some influence on your thoughts, and the more positive your thoughts are, the happier you'll feel, no matter the situation. You'll see that when you're angry, and you expressly choose instead to think a different thought (for example: What a gorgeous day it is today!), your anger will melt like snow under the sun. These are some of those little exercises that help you become conscious of these techniques. You'll be amazed at how simple this process really is. The mental exercises cannot cure your MCS, but they do make life far more pleasant, because you learn to see things through a different lens.

The following are a few books that could help you on your way. But don't forget: Use books or seminars as tools to become happier and more able to accept your current life and its limitations. Beware of "gurus" who blame you for your own MCS. We know better than that!

Empowerment: The Art of Creating Your Life As You Want It
David Gershon and Gail Straub
Empowerment Institute
234 pages

A very good practical book that thoroughly explains how to affirm, visualize and create your own happiness, and tackles all aspects of your life. It asks questions that will allow you to easily discover your points of growth, and, among other things, helps you to make your personal affirmations and visualizations. MCS patients are often constrained with regard to employment, relationships and health. This book gives you the tools with which to lead a fulfilling life.

You Can Heal Your Life
Louise L. Hay
Hay House
267 pages

A beautiful, illustrated book (different editions are available) in which the author emphasizes, among other things, how important it is to love yourself and to think positive thoughts about many issues in your life (such as your past or your body). Yet in this book she also includes a list of the possible causes of conditions and diseases which from my point of view should be taken with a sizeable grain of salt.

With this book, it's advisable to focus entirely on those things which, to you, feel like they are worthwhile to learn (working with affirmations and/or visualizations) and to disregard that which is incompatible with your impression of reality. Most of this book is worth reading; it clearly demonstrates how you can influence your own thoughts and how to train yourself to do so. After all, in order to achieve happiness we don't have to agree with everything everyone says, but they can still teach us many useful things!

Unlimited Power: The New Science of Personal Achievement

Anthony Robbins
Free Press
448 pages

In this book, Anthony Robbins explains what neuro-linguistic programming (NLP) is and what NLP can do for you. This technique is relatively easy to learn: if you visually imagine what you'd like to accomplish, then this visualization or thought has a big influence on your experiences, your actions and eventually in achieving results. The more you learn about and actually start using the ideas offered in this book, the more you start realizing that things really do work this way.

340. Spirituality

Also see *entries 89* and *290*.
These are a few wonderful spiritual books, which could well provide you with support.

The Art of Happiness: A Handbook for Living

Howard Cutler and the Dalai Lama
Riverhead Books
336 pages

Re-member: A Handbook for Human Evolution

Steve Rother
Lightworker Publications
352 pages

Conversations with God: An Uncommon Dialogue

Neale Donald Walsch
Putnam
211 pages

A Return to Love: Reflections on the Principles of "A Course in Miracles"

Marianne Williamson
Harper Paperbacks
336 pages

341. Inspirational quotes

An unbelieved truth can hurt a man much more than a lie. It takes great courage to back truth unacceptable to our times...

(John Steinbeck, *East of Eden*)

The only way to make sense out of change is to plunge into it, move with it, and join the dance.

(Alan W. Watts)

Every man has his own destiny: the only imperative is to follow it, to accept it, no matter where it leads him.

(Henry Miller)

It is not a sign of good health to be well adjusted to a sick society.

(J. Krishnamurti)

You have to accept whatever comes and the only important thing is that you meet it with courage and with the best that you have to give.

(Eleanor Roosevelt)

Absence of proof is not proof of absence.

(William Cowper)

Courage doesn't always roar. Sometimes courage is the quiet voice at the end of the day saying, "I will try again tomorrow."

(Mary Anne Radmacher)

Silence is the great revelation.

(Lao-Tse)

"The Serenity Prayer"
God grant me the serenity to accept the things I cannot change; courage to change the things I can; and wisdom to know the difference.

(Reinhold Niebuhr)

We can let the circumstances of our lives harden us so that we become increasingly resentful and afraid, or we can let them soften us, and make us kinder. We always have the choice.

(Dalai Lama)

Thank God for my handicaps, for through them, I have found myself, my work and my God.

(Helen Keller)

That which does not kill us makes us stronger.

(Friedrich Nietzsche)

The best remedy for those who are afraid, lonely or unhappy is to go outside, somewhere where they can be quiet, alone with the heavens, nature and God. Because only then does one feel that all is as
it should be and that God wishes to see people happy, amidst the simple beauty of nature.

(Anne Frank)

Just as a dew-drop on the tip of a blade of grass will quickly vanish at sunrise and will not last long; even so is the human life like a dew-drop. It is short, limited and brief. This one should wisely understand.

(Buddha)

The basic thing is that everyone wants happiness, no one wants suffering. And happiness mainly comes from our own attitude, rather than from external factors. If your own mental attitude is correct, even if you remain in a hostile atmosphere, you feel happy.

(Dalai Lama)

When one door of happiness closes, another opens; but often we look so long at the closed door that we do not see the one which has been opened for us.

(Helen Keller)

People spend a lifetime searching for happiness; looking for peace. They chase idle dreams, addictions, religions, even other people, hoping to fill the emptiness that plagues them. The irony is the only place they ever needed to search was within.

(Ramona L. Anderson)

No one can make you feel inferior without your consent.

(Eleanor Roosevelt)

Here is the test to find whether your mission on Earth is finished: if you're alive, it isn't.

(Richard Bach)

PART VI
Further Resources

18

Articles

A selection from the many articles available on www.the-abc-of-mcs.com.

342. Scientific Publications

A Cross-Sectional Study of Self-Reported Chemical-Related Sensitivity Is Associated with Gene Variants of Drug-Metabolizing Enzymes

Eckart Schnakenberg, et al.
www.ncbi.nlm.nih.gov/pubmed/172913
52?dopt=Abstract

A Review of a Two-Phase Population Study of Multiple Chemical Sensitivities

S.M. Caress and A.C. Steinemann
www.ncbi.nlm.nih.gov/pubmed/129488
89?dopt=Abstract

Bibliography of All Peer-Reviewed Scientific Papers, Official Reports, Etc.

http://mcsrr.org/resources/bibliography/

Capsaicin Inhalation Test

Ewa Ternesten
www.sffa.nu/Webbsidor/Abstract/2005_
Ewa_Ternesten.pdf

Case Report: MCS Diagnosed in a 5-Year-Old Girl

Naoko Inomata, et al.
http://ai.jsaweb.jp/fulltext/055020203/
055020203_index.html

Chemical Sensitivity Based on Biopsy Studies

William J. Meggs
www.ehponline.org/members/1997/Sup
pl-2/meggs-full.html

Definition of MCS: A 1999 Consensus

Environmental Law Centre
www.elc.org.uk/pages/healthmcsdefiniti
on.htm

Definition of MCS: Case Definitions for Multiple Chemical Sensitivity

Nicholas A. Ashford and Claudia S. Miller
http://books.nap.edu/openbook.php?is
bn=0309047366&page=41

Definition of MCS: Toward a Working Case Definition

J.R. Nethercott, et al.
www.ncbi.nlm.nih.gov/pubmed/84523
95?dopt=Abstract

Effect of Prolonged Exposure to Low Concentrations of Formaldehyde on the Corticotropin-Releasing Hormone Neurons in the Hypothalamus and Adrenocorticotropic Hormone Cells in the Pituitary Gland in Female Mice

D.K. Sari, et al.
www.ncbi.nlm.nih.gov/pubmed/151969
73?dopt=AbstractPlus

Elevated Nitric Oxide/Peroxynitrite Theory of Multiple Chemical Sensitivity: Central Role of N-methyl-D-aspartate Receptors in the Sensitivity Mechanism
Martin L. Pall
www.pubmedcentral.nih.gov/articleren der.fcgi?artid=1241647

Environmental Project no. 988, 2005: Multiple Chemical Sensitivity (MCS)
www2.mst.dk/Udgiv/publications/ 2005/87-7614-548-4/html/helepubl_ eng.htm

Environmentally Triggered Disorders
W. J. Rea
www.aehf.com/articles/A19.htm

Exposure to Repeated Low-Level Formaldehyde in Rats Increases Basal Corticosterone Levels and Enhances the Corticosterone Response to Subsequent Formaldehyde
B.A. Sorg, et al.
www.ncbi.nlm.nih.gov/pubmed/113060 18?dopt=AbstractPlus

Neurotoxicity in Single Photon Emission Computed Tomography Brain Scans of Patients Reporting Chemical Sensitivities
G.H. Ross, et al.
www.ncbi.nlm.nih.gov/pubmed/104162 94?dopt=AbstractPlus

Odor Sensitivity and Respiratory Complaint Profiles in a Community-Based Sample with Asthma, Hay Fever, and Chemical Odor Intolerance
C.M. Baldwin, et al.
www.ncbi.nlm.nih.gov/pubmed/104162 92?dopt=Abstract

Prevalence of Multiple Chemical Sensitivities: A Population-Based Study in the Southeastern United States
Stanley M. Caress and Anne C. Steinemann
www.pubmedcentral.nih.gov/articleren der.fcgi?tool=pubmed&pubmedid= 15117694

Profile of Patients with MCS
Grace Ziem and James McTamney
www.mindfully.org/Health/Profile-Patients-MCS.htm

Symptom Profile of Multiple Chemical Sensitivity in Actual Life
M. Saito, et al.
www.ncbi.nlm.nih.gov/pubmed/157848 00?dopt=Abstract

The Problems of MCS Patients in Using Medicinal Drugs
J. Suzuki, et al.
www.ncbi.nlm.nih.gov/pubmed/152977 26?dopt=Abstract

Toxicant-Induced Loss of Tolerance
Claudia S. Miller
www.herc.org/news/ehp/miller.html

343. Magazine and Website Articles

Biomarkers of MCS
www.mcsrr.org/resources/biomarkers.ht ml

Case-Control Study of Genotypes in Multiple Chemical Sensitivity
G. McKeown-Eyssen, et al.
www.protectingourhealth.org/newsci ence/immune/2004/2004–0715mcke own-eyssenetal.htm

Defining Chemical Injury: Diagnostic Protocol

G. Heuser, et al.

www.iicph.org/docs/ipph_Defining_Ch
   emical_Injury.htm

Engaging with MCS

Malcolm Hooper

www.satori-5.co.uk/word_articles/
   mcs/engaging_with_mcs.html

Multiple Chemical Sensitivities under Siege

Ann McCampbell

www.getipm.com/personal/mcs-
   campbell.htm

Multiple Chemical Sensitivity: Towards the End of Controversy

Martin L. Pall

http://findarticles.com/p/articles/mi_m0
   ISW/is_265–266/ai_n15688810/pg_1

344. Miscellaneous Articles

Interview with Rosalind Anderson

www.exposed.at/anderson.htm

Dr. Grace Ziem's Environmental Control Plan for MCS Patients

www.mcsrr.org/resources/articles/S3.ht
   ml

MCS: What It Is, What It Is Not and How It Is Manifested

http://users.lmi.net/wilworks/newreact/
   sbastien.htm

Multiple Chemical Sensitivities: Facts, Fiction, Disability and the Law

Gail Sullivan Restivo

www.lectlaw.com/filesh/csl01.htm

Multiple Chemical Sensitivities Information Sheet and Selected References

Mark Donohoe

http://homepage.mac.com/doctormark/
   Acrobat/MCS/MCS_info_refs.pdf

Perceived Treatment Efficacy for Conventional and Alternative Therapies Reported by Persons with MCS

Pamela Reed Gibson, Amy Nicole-
   Marie Elms, and Lisa Ann Ruding

www.ehponline.org/members/2003/
   5936/5936.html

Psychogenic Origins of Multiple Chemical Sensitivities Syndrome: A Critical Review of the Research Literature

Ann L. Davidoff, Linda Fogarty

www.ncbi.nlm.nih.gov/sites/entrez?cmd
   =Retrieve&db=PubMed&list_uids=7
   944561&dopt=Citation

Recognition of MCS As a Disability by the U.S. Department of Housing and Urban Development (HUD) and the Social Security Administration (SSA)

www.ed.gov/policy/speced/guid/rsa/im/
   2002/im-02–04.pdf

19

Websites

Warning: not every product or link mentioned is suitable for every MCS patient. Cautious testing and/or outgassing is required !!

This chapter contains a list of relevant online addresses that was accurate as of this writing. For a complete and continuously updated list, go to www.-the-abc-of-mcs.com.

345. Air Pollution

Air Fresheners (or "Air Poisoners"?) YOU Decide!!
www.ourlittleplace.com/air.html

Air Now: Local Air Quality Conditions and Forecasts
http://cfpub.epa.gov/airnow/index.cfm?action=airnow.main

American Lung Association: State of the Air
www.stateoftheair.org

The Cleaner Indoor Campaign
www.cleanerindoorair.org

ESA Portal: Global Air Pollution
www.esa.int/esaCP/SEM340NKPZD_index_0.html

Scorecard, The Pollution Information Site
www.scorecard.org

SSD Fire Detection Program
www.firedetect.noaa.gov/viewer.htm

346. Air Purifiers

AllerAir:
http://allerair.com/
www.allerair.com/air-purifiers/air-purifiers-home-office-multiple-chemical-sensitivity.html
www.achooallergy.com/allerair-airmedic-mcs-mscd-airpurifiers.asp

Amaircare Roomaid:
www.achooallergy.com/roomaid.asp
www.allergyasthmatech.com/P/Amaircare_Roomaid/593_315

Austin Air:
http://austinair.com
www.achooallergy.com/austinhealthmate-superblend.asp

General links on air purifying:
www.achooallergy.com/mcs-air-quality.asp
www.home-air-purifier-expert.com/index.html

IQair:
www.iqair.com/EU/ENG/Products/GC Series.htm
www.achooallergy.com/iqairpurifiers.asp
http://www.achooallergy.com/IQAIR GCGCX.asp

Portable ionizer:
www.natlallergy.com/product.asp?pn=1121&bhcd2=1225104378
www.negativeiongenerators.com/portableairpurifier.html

Powered Air Purifying Respirator (PAPR):

www.3m.com

www.msanorthamerica.com/catalog/catalog526.html

www.safetycompany.com/powered-air-purifying-respirator-powered-air-purifying-respira/c_13_230_231.html?osCsid=801a7cbd01d5f1ae6c1a61ae3712169f

347. Allergies (Products)

Be careful, allergy products are not MCS products! For specific MCS products go to *entry 373* "Products online."

Allergy Buyers Club
www.allergybuyersclub.com/index.html

Allergy Control Products
www.allergycontrol.com

Allergy Relief Store
http://onlineallergyrelief.com/index.html

Allergy Store
www.allergystore.com

National Allergy
www.natlallergy.com

348. Asthma and Allergy

American Lung Association
www.lungusa.org

Asthma and Allergy Foundation of America
www.aafa.org

349. Building Materials

PAINTS AND PRODUCTS

www.afmsafecoat.com

www.bioshieldpaint.com

www.eartheasy.com/live_nontoxic_paints.htm

www.eco-house.com

www.ecospaints.com

www.milkpaint.com

www.naturalhomeproducts.com

www.natureneutral.com

RECYCLING

www.neo.ne.gov/home_const/factsheets/recycled_const_mat.htm

RESOURCE LISTS

www.lassentech.com/eibuld.html

www.planetthrive.com/members/PDFs/Safer%20Construction%20Tips%20read%20only.pdf

http://yellowcanary.com/build_green

350. Chemicals and Toxins

DRY CLEANING WITHOUT HARMFUL CHEMICALS

www.naturalnews.com/023365.html

www.drycleaningstation.com

RELATION BETWEEN CHEMICALS AND HEALTH

The Collaborative on Health and the Environment Database http://database.healthandenvironment.org/index.cfm

Relational database of Hazardous Chemicals and Occupational Diseases www.haz-map.com

MISCELLANEOUS

Material Safety Data Sheets (MSDS) Databases www.msdssearch.com/DBLinksN.htm

REACH (law in Europe on chemical safety/registration): http://ec.europa.eu/environment/chemicals/reach/reach_intro.htm; www.chemicalspolicy.org/downloads/REACHisHere220307.pdf

351. Clothing

Blue Canoe Organic Cotton Clothing
www.bluecanoe.com

Cotton Field USA
www.cottonfieldusa.com

Kasper Organics
www.kasperorganics.com

Lotus Organics
http://lotusorganics.com

Maggie's Functional Organics
www.maggiesorganics.com

No Pity Shirts
http://nopityshirts.com

The Oko Box
www.theokobox.com

Rawganique
www.rawganique.com

Truly organic
www.truly-organic.com/shop/home.php

Wildlife Works
www.wildlifeworks.com

Zona's T-Shirts & Stuff Zone
http://members.shaw.ca/zonaszone/shop/tshirts.html

352. Dental

The Dentist Referral List by State of MCS-America:
http://mcs-america.org/dentistlist.pdf

Stason.org (dental information for the chemically sensitive patient)
http://stason.org/TULARC/health/dental-amalgam/13-Is-There-Information-For-The-Chemically-Sensitive-Patient.html

Toxic Teeth: Consumers for Dental Choice
www.toxicteeth.org

353. Doctors, Physicians and Therapists

American Academy of Environmental Medicine
www.aaemonline.org

American College of Occupational and Environmental Medicine
www.acoem.org

American Holistic Medical Association
www.holisticmedicine.org

Association of Occupational and Environmental Clinics
www.aoec.org

Doctors Treating MCS and/or CFS/FM Nationwide
http://mcs-america.org/doctorlist.pdf

Doris J. Rapp, M.D.
www.drrapp.com

Gunnar Heuser, M.D., Ph.D., F.A.C.P
www.toxgun.com

See also *entry 355*, "Environmental Health Center."

354. EMF and Protection/ Out-Gassing Computers

EMF Pollution FAQs
www.toolsforhealing.com/products/EM
FProducts/Articles/FAQs.html

EMR-EMF (an open mailing list for the discussion of electromagnetic radiation)
http://groups.yahoo.com/group/emr-emf/

Energy Fields
www.energyfields.org

Low-emission computers
www.asilo.com/aztap1

Mockia — strange telecom (radiation free horns for cell phones)
www.mockia.com/store.html

The Outgas Report (information about out-gassed chemicals from computers and other sources)
www.outgasreport.com/index.html

Technology Alternatives Corporation: Non-Chemical Radiation-Free Computers
www.safelevel.com/index.html

Weep: Living with EHS
www.weepinitiative.org/livingwith
EHS.html

355. Environmental Health Centers

Breakspear Hospital, England
www.breakspearmedical.com

Center For Occupational and Environmental Medicine
http://coem.com

Environmental Health Center
www.ehcd.com

The Environmental Health Center at the Woman's College Hospital, Canada
www.womenshealthmatters.ca/Centres/
environmental/

Johnson Medical Associates
www.johnsonmedicalassociates.com

The Nova Scotia Environmental Health Centre, Canada
www.cdha.nshealth.ca

Robbins' Environmental Medicine Center
http://allergycenter.com

Also see *entry 353* "Doctors, Physicians and Therapists."

356. Environmental Organizations

Californians for Alternatives to Toxics
www.alternatives2toxics.org

The Cleaner Indoor Air Campaign
www.cleanerindoorair.org

Envirolink: The Online Environmental Community
www.envirolink.org

Environmental Defense Fund
www.edf.org/home.cfm

Environmental Directories Online
www.ulb.ac.be/ceese/meta/cds.html

Environmental Health Coalition
www.environmentalhealth.org

Environmental Working Group
www.ewg.org

Friends of the Earth
www.foe.org

Greenpeace USA
www.greenpeace.org/usa

Human Ecology Action League, Inc. (HEAL)
www.healnatl.org/index.html

Natural Resources Defense Council
www.nrdc.org

Toxic Nation Canada
http://toxicnation.ca

Washington Toxics Coalition
www.watoxics.org

357. Forums

GENERAL LINKS

Directory of Yahoo MCS groups
http://health.dir.groups.yahoo.com/dir/ 1603388362

GROUPS IN ALPHABETICAL ORDER

Chemical Injury Support
http://health.groups.yahoo.com/group/c hemicalinjurysupport

CMCS-EI: Christians with Invisible Illnesses
http://health.groups.yahoo.com/group/ CMCS-EI

Creative Canaries Community
http://health.groups.yahoo.com/group/ CreativeCanariesCommunity

Green Canary
http://groups.yahoo.com/group/Green Canary

MCS Canada
http://health.groups.yahoo.com/group/ MCS-Canada

MCS Canadian Sources
http://groups.yahoo.com/group/MCS-CanadianSources

MCS-International: The Sanctuary
www.mcs-international.org/phpBB3

MCS Photography
http://health.groups.yahoo.com/group/ MCSphotography

MCS Recycle
http://groups.yahoo.com/group/MCSR ecycle

MCS Safe Shelter USA
http://health.groups.yahoo.com/group/ mcssafeshelterusa

MCS Writers Group
http://health.groups.yahoo.com/group/ mcswritersgroup

Planet Thrive
www.planetthrive.com

358. Furniture

Nirvana Safe Haven
www.nontoxic.com/organicfurniture/ch emicalfreeseating.html

Organic furniture
http://furnature.com/index.html

359. Government

Environmental Protection Agency
www.epa.gov

National Institute of Environmental Health Sciences
www.niehs.nih.gov

National Institute for Occupational Safety and Health
www.cdc.gov/NIOSH/

National Institutes of Health (NIH)
www.nih.gov

Social Security Online
www.ssa.gov

U.S. Consumer Product Safety Commission
www.cpsc.gov

U.S. Department of Housing and Urban Development
www.hud.gov

U.S. Department of Justice — Americans with Disabilities Act
www.ada.gov

U.S. Food and Drug Administration
www.fda.gov

World Health Organization
www.who.int/en/

360. Hospital

Hospitalization for the Chemical Sensitive Patient
www.citlink.net/~bhima/hospital.htm

MCS Canadian Sources: Hospital Protocols
www.mscanadian.org/hospital.html

MCS hospital access
www.healsoaz.org/hospital_access.htm

Tips for Anesthetics and Hospitalization for People with Multiple Chemical Sensitivities
www.immuneweb.org/articles/anesthetics.html

361. Housing and Living

MCS HOUSING

CIIN — MCS housing
www.ciin.org/pages/09-housing.html

E Magazine "No Safe Haven: People with Multiple Chemical Sensitivity Are Becoming the New Homeless"
www.emagazine.com/view/?1003

Ecology House Rules
www.tikvah.com/cc/eh/ruleslists.html

Ecology House, San Rafael, California
www.tikvah.com/cc/eh/

Environmental Health Association of Ontario (7 units for the chemical sensitive)
http://ehaontario.ca/barrhaven-housing.htm

Quail Haven — MCS Housing
http://madelinx.tripod.com/
http://dianeensign.tripod.com/index.html

Seagonville Ecology Housing (only for patients of www.ehcd.com)
www.ehcd.com/websteen/seagoville.htm

Tad Taylor's Healthy Homes
www.healthy-homes.com/

Yahoo group about short-term and long-term housing for people with MCS
http://health.groups.yahoo.com/group/mcssafeshelterusa

GENERAL INFORMATION ON GREEN LIVING

Architectural House Plans
www.architecturalhouseplans.com/healthy_homes/

Green HHHomes for Sale
http://greenhomesforsale.com

Healthy House Institute
www.healthyhouseinstitute.com

International Institute for Bau Biologie (a movement promoting healthy building principles)
www.buildingbiology.net

Safe Homes (environmental consultants)
http://safe-homes.com

MCS INFO FROM THE HEALTHY HOUSING COALITION

Basic Needs for Rental Housing for Chemically Sensitive Persons
www.herc.org/hhc/Basicrentalneeds.html

MCS and Less Toxic Living
www.herc.org/hhc/MCSfactfict.html

MCS Living in New Mexico
www.herc.org/hhc/NMAreaMCSInfo.html

Safe Housing Tips: What to Look For in an Existing House for a Healthier Home
www.herc.org/hhc/What2Look4.html

LINK LISTS

www.princesstigerlily.com/mcs/housing.html
http://mcs-america.org/EnvironmentalIllnessMCSSupportandReosurces.htm#_Housing_Resources_and

362. Laboratories

Accu-Chem Laboratories
www.accuchem.com

Anderson Laboratories
www.andersonlaboratories.com
    See also an interview at: www.exposed.at/anderson.htm

Doctor's Data Inc.
www.doctorsdata.com

Genova Diagnostics
www.genovadiagnostics.com

Indoor Air Surveys
www.IndoorAirSurveys.com

363. Legal

Environment and human rights advisory
www.environmentandhumanrights.org

Environmental lawyers
www.environmentallawyers.com

MCS Advocacy
http://mcsadvocacy.org/

MCS Beacon of Hope: Legal Links, Cases and Information:
www.mcsbeaconofhope.com/MCS%20BOH/legal_links.htm

MCS legal help
http://mcslegalhelp.com

MCS survivors: legal aid (resource list)
http://mcsurvivors.com/dcd/Legal_Aid/

Multiple Chemical Sensitivity: Recognition to Proof: Thelma S. Cohen,

Esq. Bertram L. Potter, Esq. Gary J. Shima, M.D.
www.disabilitylawcentral.com/index page_6/Articles.shtml

National Network of ADA Centers (Americans with Disabilities Act)
www.adata.org

364. Masks/Respirators

MCS ORGANIC COTTON MASKS

The American Environmental Health Foundation (AEHF)
www.aehf.com

I Can Breathe! Masks
http://icanbreathe.com/

Nutritional Ecological Environmental Delivery System (NEEDS)
www.needs.com

POWERED AIR PURIFYING RESPIRATOR (PAPR)

www.3m.com
www.msanorthamerica.com/catalog/cat alog526.html
www.westernsafety.com/3m/3mrespi ratorypg4.html
www.safetycompany.com/powered-air-purifying-respirator-powered-air-puri fying-respira/c_13_230_231.html ?osCsid=801a7cbd01d5flae6c1a61ae3 712169f

GENERAL LINKS ON SAFETY SUPPLIES/MASKS

www.msanorthamerica.com/catalog/cat alog503.html

www.labsafety.com/store/Safety_Sup plies/Respirators/Air-Purifying_ Respirators/?recsPerPage=45
www.respro.com
www.websoft-solutions.net/protective_ respirators_safety_respirators_s/42. htm
www.westernsafety.com/resppro.htm

365. Mattresses, Bedding and More

The Clean Bedroom
www.thecleanbedroom.com

EcoChoices Natural Living Store
www.ecochoices.com

Heart of Vermont
www.heartofvermont.com

Janice's
http://janices.com

Lifekind
www.lifekind.com

Nirvana Safe Haven
www.nirvanasafehaven.com

Satara, Inc.
www.satara-inc.com

Tomorrow's World
www.tomorrowsworld.com

366. MCS organizations

The Chemical Injury Information Network (CIIN)
www.ciin.org

Chemical Injury.Net
www.chemicalinjury.net/index.htm

The Chemical Sensitivity Foundation
www.chemicalsensitivityfoundation.
  org

Creative Canaries
www.creativecanaries.org

Environmental Health Network
http://users.lmi.net/wilworks/

The Environmental Illness Resource
www.ei-resource.org

MCS-America
www.mcs-america.org

The MCS Beacon of Hope
www.mcsbeaconofhope.com

MCS Global
www.mcs-global.org

MCS International
www.mcs-international.org

MCS Referral & Resources
www.mcsrr.org

Planet Thrive
www.planetthrive.com

The Rocky Mountain Environmental
  Health Association
http://bcn.boulder.co.us/health/rmeha/i
  ndex.htm

Lists of MCS websites/organizations:
www.princesstigerlily.com/mcs/mcs_by
  _area.html

367. Miscellaneous

ART AND/OR HUMOR

www.cafepress.com/buy/canary/multi
  ple+chemical+sensitivity
www.cafepress.com/zonas_mcs

www.citlink.net/~bhima/artists.htm
www.creativecanaries.org
www.planetthrive.com
www.sickhumorpostcards.com
http://health.groups.yahoo.com/group/
  CreativeCanariesCommunity
http://toxicamenders.googlepages.com/
  toxicamenderse-greetingcards

BIONASE

www.intelligenthealthsystems.com.au/bi
  onase.htm
www.smartmiracles.com/p-Gifts-75-
  100/BS511/Bionase+Nasal+Applicator.
  html

ELECTRONIC CANDLES

www.norexbuydirect.com

HEALTHY CARS

www.healthycar.org/home.php

MOLD

www.moldacrossamerica.org

NOSE FILTERS

www.nosefilters.com/prod01.htm

OXYGEN

www.aehf.com/catalog/product_info.ph
  p?products_id=916
www.emergencypax.com/oxygen/
www.open-aire.com

PETS

http://naturalanimal.com

READING BOXES

http://mcsinfo.homestead.com/reading

box.html http://au.geocities.com/dj_
ludlow/mcs/readboxintro.pdf

SAFER CHOICES

www.eartheasy.com/live_nontoxic_solu
tions.htm
www.ecologycenter.org/factsheets/clean
ing.html
www.lesstoxicguide.ca/index.asp
www.mcsbeaconofhope.com/safercho
ices.html

TRI-SALTS

www.absolutelythepurest.com/suppleme
nts/Tri%20Salts.html
www.needs.com/product/Ecological_Fo
rmulas_Tri_Salts_200/vspgb_Ecologi
cal_Formulas
http://store.agoodvitamin.com/ecfotr
200mg.html

TYVEK COVERALLS

www.abcsafetymart.com/clothing/cloth
ing.html
www.tasco-safety.com/tyvek-protective-
clothing.html

368. Organic

Eco Mall
www.ecomall.com

Eco Planet
www.ecoplanet.com

Organic Consumers Association
www.organicconsumers.org

ORGANIC FLOWERS

www.localharvest.org/organic-flowers.jsp
www.ecobusinesslinks.com/organic_flo
wers.htm

ORGANIC HAIR SALONS

http://hair.lovetoknow.com/Aveda_Org
anic_Hair_Salon
www.johnmasters.com/salon.htm
www.ecocolors.net/

ORGANIC/NATURAL PRINTING

www.naturalprinting.net
www.naturalprinting.com
www.naturalsourceprinting.com

The Organic Pages
www.theorganicpages.com/topo/index.h
tml

Planet Organics
www.planetorganics.com

Trader Joe's
www.traderjoes.com

Whole Foods Supermarket
www.wholefoodsmarket.com/products/

Also see *entry 373* "Products online."

369. Overlapping Diseases

CFS (CHRONIC FATIGUE SYNDROME)

CFIDS Association of America
www.cfids.org

Co-Cure Myalgic Encephalomyelitis/
Chronic Fatigue Syndrome (ME/
CFS) and Fibromyalgia
www.co-cure.org

Diagnosing CFS
www.cdc.gov/cfs/pdf/Diagnosing_CFS.p
df
www.cdc.gov/cfs/cfssymptomsHCP.htm
(symptoms including MCS)

FIBROMYALGIA

American Fibromyalgia Syndrome Association
www.afsafund.org

Fibromyalgia Coalition International
www.fibrocoalition.org

Fibromyalgia Information Foundation
www.myalgia.com

Fibromyalgia Network
www.fmnetnews.com

National Fibromyalgia Association
www.fmaware.org

GULF WAR SYNDROME

American Gulf War Veterans Association
www.gulfwarvets.com

Desert Storm Justice Foundation:
www.dsjf.org

Gulf War Veteran Resource Page
www.gulfweb.org

SICK BUILDING SYNDROME

Indoor Air Facts No. 4 (Revised) Sick Building Syndrome
www.epa.gov/iaq/pubs/sbs.html

Sick Building Syndrome Modern Day Dilemma
www.home-air-purifier-expert.com/sick-building-syndrome.html

Sick Building Syndrome (SBS)
www.ei-resource.org/illness-information/related-conditions/sick-building-syndrome-(sbs)/

GENERAL

Read more about CFS, MCS and overlapping diseases:
www.satori-5.co.uk/word_articles/mcs/engaging_with_mcs.html

370. Perfume-free

Campaign for fragrance-free health care in the U.S.
www.massnurses.org/health/articles/chemexpos0406_1.htm

Canada Safety Council — Perfume in the Workplace
www.safety-council.org/info/OSH/perfume.html

Canadian Centre for Occupational Health and Safety Scent-Free Policy for the Workplace
www.ccohs.ca/oshanswers/hsprograms/scent_free.html

Chemical Awareness in Schools
www.netspeed.com.au/rdi/cas/aboutus.html

Health Care without Harm
www.noharm.org/us/pesticidesCleaners/Fragrances

Health Risks from Perfume: The Most Common Chemicals Found in Thirty-One Fragrance Products
http://immuneweb.org/articles/perfume.html

No Fragrance.org
http://nofragrance.org/

No Scents Make Sense — The Lung Association of Canada
www.nb.lung.ca/pdf/NoScentsMakeSense.pdf

Scientific Instrument Services, Inc. The Analysis of Perfumes and Their Effect on Indoor Air Pollution
www.sisweb.com/referenc/applnote/app-73i.htm

371. Personal Care

Also see *entry 373*, "Products online."

All Natural Cosmetics
www.allnaturalcosmetics.com

Aubreyorganics
www.aubrey-organics.com

Canary Cosmetics
www.canarycosmetics.com

Real Purity
www.realpurity.com

Sungold Soap
www.sungoldsoap.com

MENSTRUAL PADS AND TAMPONS

www.alyahs.com/SearchResults.asp?Cat=3
www.hankettes.com/qs/product/8/153/143455/0/0
http://manymoonsalternatives.com/category.php?cat_id=9
www.natracare.com
www.organiccottonplus.com/mp.html

372. Pesticides

The Best Control: Intelligent Pest Management
www.thebestcontrol.com

Beyond Pesticides: National Coalition against the Misuse of Pesticides
www.beyondpesticides.org

Biocontrol Network
www.biconet.com

Nature's Best Indoor Pest Control
www.maskedflowerimages.com/pestcontrol.html

Nature's Best Outdoor Pest Control
www.maskedflowerimages.com/nontoxicpestcontrol.htm

No Spray Coalition
www.nospray.org

Safe Solutions Sustainable Living & Natural Home Products
www.safesolutionsinc.com

373. Products Online

PARTLY MCS-ORIENTED PRODUCTS

American Environmental Health Foundation (AEHF) (Founded by dr. Rea, director of www.ehcd.com)
www.aehf.com

National Ecological and Environmental Delivery System (N.E.E.D.S.)
www.needs.com

FOOD

Diamond Organics (fresh organic meals)
www.diamondorganics.com

Organic Foods Online
http://organicfoodcart.com

Body, Food, Health and
Home (Not Specifically
MCS-Oriented):

Health Goods
www.healthgoods.com

Organic Kingdom
www.organickingdom.com

Shop Organic
www.shoporganic.com

Also see *entry 369*, "Organic."

374. Religion and Spirituality

Aroma of Christ Ministry
www.aromaofchrist.com

Free Meditations — Techniques for Positive Thinking and Meditation
www.freemeditations.com

Holistic Online (about alternative therapies, meditation, spirituality)
http://holisticonline.com

Share, Care and Prayer, Inc.
www.sharecareprayer.org

Where Is God Ministries: Why Go Perfume-Free to Church? Accessibility for the Chemically Sensitive
www.whereisgod.net/pfchurch.htm

Yahoo Internet Group: CMCS-EI: Christians with Invisible Illnesses
http://health.groups.yahoo.com/group/CMCS-EI

375. Saunas

SAUNA SPECIALLY BUILT
FOR MCS PATIENTS

Green Living Oasis Heavenly Heat Saunas
www.greenlivingoasis.com/saunas.html

Heavenly Heat Saunas — Bob Morgan
www.heavenlyheatsaunas.com

INFORMATION ON BUILDING
YOUR OWN SAUNA

www.drlwilson.com/Articles/sauna_therapy.htm
http://drlwilson.com/Books/saunabook.htm

SAUNAS, NOT SPECIFICALLY
BUILT FOR MCS PATIENTS

High Tech Health
www.hightechhealth.com

Saunafin Saunas and Steambaths
www.saunafin.com

Soft Heat Saunas,
www.infraredsauna.net

Sunlight Saunas
www.sunlightsaunas.com

376. Schools/Children

The Center for School Mold Help
www.schoolmoldhelp.org

The Green Flag program
www.greenflagschools.org

Healthy Child, Healthy World
http://healthychild.org

Healthy Schools Network, Inc.
www.healthyschools.org

377. Stories of MCS Patients

Aroma of Christ: Faces of the Chemically Sensitive
www.aromaofchrist.com/Faces%20of%20MCS%20Title%20Page.htm

Chemical Illness Report Page
www.chem-tox.com/guest-whistle/guestbook.html

Gathering Stories about Chemical Injury
www.citlink.net/~bhima/gathering.htm

MCS-International: Meet the Team
www.mcs-international.org/about_us/meet_the_team.html

"No Safe Haven: People with MCS Are Becoming the New Homeless"
www.emagazine.com/view/?1003

Personal stories from MCS patients around the EHC — Dallas
www.ehcd.com/websteen/ehcd_patient_stories.htm

Read these people's stories, then consider this, could you be next?
www.mcs-global.org/Stories.htm

Share a day in your life with chronic illness
http://planetthrive.com/cgi-bin/members/pub9990215236064.cgi

The wall of personal testimony
www.herc.org/wall

378. Travel

Flying with disability
www.flying-with-disability.org

MCS Travel
http://mcstravel.resourcez.com

MCS Travel Directory
www.safertraveldirectory.com

The Natural Place — Florida Environmental Residence and Hotel for People with MCS
www.thenaturalplace.com

Yahoo group: MCS Safe Shelter USA — Short-term and long-term housing for people with MCS
http://health.groups.yahoo.com/group/mcssafeshelterusa/

Yellow Canary — Environmentally Safe Travel
http://yellowcanary.com/travelsafe/

379. Video/Movies

Chemical Injury.Net (Dr. Ziem)
www.chemicalinjury.net/videosandmedia.htm

Chemical Kids
www.mediarights.org/film/chemical_kids
www.filmakers.com/index.php?a=filmDetail&filmID=1053

Chemical Sensitivity: A 15-Minute Introduction (Chemical Sensitivity Foundation)
www.chemicalsensitivityfoundation.org/chemical-sensitivity-introduction-15-minute.htm

Exposed
www.exposed.at

Final Insult
www.roninfilms.com.au/video/1871977/0/1832141.html

Funny, You Don't Look Sick (Susan Abod)
www.susanabod.com/funny.html

Homesick trailer (Susan Abod)
www.homesick-video.com

MCS: How Chemical Exposures May Be Affecting Your Health (Alison Johnson)
www.alisonjohnsonmcs.com

[SAFE] (Todd Haynes)
www.sonypictures.com/classics/safe/safe.html

The Toxic Clouds of 9/11: A Looming Health Disaster
www.alisonjohnsonmcs.com/toxic-clouds-911-dvd-trailer.htm?v=6aolE1i486w

380. Water

American Environmental Health Foundation (AEHF)
www.aehf.com (see water filters)

Home Water Purification Systems
www.cleanairpurewater.com

National Ecological and Environmental Delivery System (N.E.E.D.S.)
www.needs.com (see water purifiers)

The Pure Water Place
www.purewaterplace.com

Shower Filter Store
www.showerfilterstore.com

381. Workplace

Canadian Human Rights Commission:
www.chrc-ccdp.ca/pdf/envsensitivity_en.pdf

PART VII

Providing Information to Others

This informational brochure about MCS is double-sided and can certainly, with permission from the author and the publisher, be reproduced for distribution many times over. It contains basic and necessary information about MCS and serves as an introduction to the disease. The aim is to stimulate the recipient to further study the subject and/or enable the recipient to be considerate of the patient. This brochure can also be downloaded at www.the-abc-of-mcs.com (click on the book cover image).

TIP

• Aside from distributing folders and possibly having people read this book, another good idea is to inform people using the documentaries that have come out on this subject. See *Part V: Films, Books and Other Resources*. The documentary *MCS: How Chemical Exposures May Be Affecting Your Health* by Alison Johnson (see *entry 321*) is also a very good place to start learning about MCS.

MCS Handout

www.the-abc-of-mcs.com

You are receiving this handout from somebody who would like to inform you about the environmental illness MCS.

If you are holding this folder in your hands, there is in all likelihood somebody in your neighborhood who has MCS or simply would like to inform you of the existence of MCS. If you are receiving this information from an MCS patient, the reason is likely that this person wants to ask for your understanding. Due to the complexity of the environmental illness MCS, it's important for people to be able to imagine what MCS is before they might misjudge an MCS patient or the disease itself.

• *What is MCS?* MCS stands for *multiple chemical sensitivity*. People who suffer from this condition get sick from all sorts of everyday (synthetic) chemical substances and/or scents. Many cannot lead normal lives because these substances are found almost everywhere. These chemically sensitive people get sick from chemical substances, even low doses to which healthy people do not display any noticeable reaction and might not even know are there.

• *Various triggers* can cause MCS to develop. At the moment, the best-known causes are: long-term (over many years) exposure to a "cocktail" of various, often low doses of chemical substances and/or a one-time exposure to a high dose of chemical substances, such as formaldehyde, solvents, pesticides, insecticides, toluene, liquid narcotics and other chemical substances. Two examples are 9/11 rescue workers and Gulf War veterans.

• An MCS patient can get sick from **many chemical substances** found in the following products (among others): laundry and cleaning detergents, personal care products, all perfume-containing products, cigarette and cigar smoke, medicine, car exhaust, pesticides/insecticides, air fresheners, new construction materials, new furniture, new carpeting, smoke and/or combustion fumes from fireplaces, furnaces or barbecues, newspapers, books, plastics and rubber, and smog/fine particles.

• The *symptoms* displayed by an MCS patient after exposure to a harmful substance are (among others): respiratory and lung problems, blackouts, chronic fatigue, lack of concentration, flu-like symptoms, cardiac arrhythmia, headaches, skin rashes, seizures, disorientation, problems with short-term memory, infections, symptoms of poisoning (nausea, shivering, dizziness, the feeling of having a hangover), and ear, nose, throat and sinus problems. Not every MCS patient displays the same symptoms. It is impossible to mention the wide range of symptoms in this brochure.

If you yourself are not an MCS patient and you have received this handout, you could perhaps help get MCS more widely recognized by learning more about MCS and the consequences it holds for MCS patients. You could, for example, be sympathetic on a number of issues or at least be considerate of the sensitivity. Living with a chemical sensitivity is no easy thing in a society awash with chemicals. Every MCS patient can use the support of family, friends, colleagues, neighbors, and doctors.

Did you know?

• Did you know perfume used to be made of flower extracts and natural animal musk, while nowadays perfumes consist of 95 percent petrochemicals? Just a fraction of the chemicals used in perfumes have been tested, and even chemicals that have been found to be toxic are still in use. Chemicals found in perfume are also found in gasoline and cigarette smoke.

• Did you know that many chemical substances in everyday consumer products, including in our food and beverages, were never tested? And that the health effects of the many chemical substances in various household and home products are still unknown? These lack of testing puts people — especially children — in danger of getting ill.

• Did you know that the existence of MCS has been identified since the 1950s? The reason it is taking so long for MCS to be completely globally recognized (though in some countries it has been partially recognized), has to do with many issues, including the complexity of the disease (it is a multi-system condition), the diverging scientific explanatory models, and the various political, economic and industrial interests that are involved.

Where can I find more information about MCS?

The book *Understanding Multiple Chemical Sensitivity* contains a great deal of information on this condition, such as tips for patients and those near to them, experiences and stories of other MCS patients, and clear explanations for doctors, therapists, students or researchers. See www.the-abc-of-mcs.com for more information on the content of this book. On this site you will also find many links to thoroughly informative American and international websites.

Thank you for reading this information!

This MCS handout may be copied and distributed to others.
This helps foster awareness of MCS, which hopefully will
engender more sympathy and understanding for
this misunderstood environmental illness.

Bibliography

Barta, L., et al. "Multiple Chemical Sensitivity (MCS): A 1999 Consensus." *Archives of Environmental Health* May–June 1999; 54(3): 147–149. www.elc.org.uk/pages/healthmcsdefinition.htm.

The Canadian Lung Association. "No Scents Make Sense." http://www.nb.lung.ca/pdf/NoScentsMakeSense.pdf.

Caress, S.M., Steinemann, A.C. "A Review of a Two-Phase Population Study of Multiple Chemical Sensitivities." *Environmental Health Perspectives* September 2003; 111(12): 1490–1497. www.ncbi.nlm.nih.gov/pubmed/12948889?dopt=Abstract.

Carter Batiste, Linda. "How to Determine Whether a Person Has a Disability under the Americans with Disabilities Act (ADA)." Job Accommodation Network, Volume 2, Issue 4, September 2008. www.jan.wvu.edu/corner/vol02iss04.htm.

Danish Environmental Protection. "Environmental Project No. 988, 2005 — Multiple Chemical Sensitivity." Version 1.0, Copenhagen, Denmark, March 2005. http://www2.mst.dk/Udgiv/publications/2005/87-7614-548-4/html/helepubl_eng.htm.

Davidoff, A.L., Fogarty, L. "Psychogenic Origins of Multiple Chemical Sensitivities Syndrome: A Critical Review of the Research Literature." *Archives of Environmental Health* September–October 1994; 49(5): 316–325. www.ncbi.nlm.nih.gov/sites/entrez?cmd=Retrieve&db=PubMed&list_uids=7944561&dopt=Citation.

Donnay, Albert H. "Bibliography of All Peer-Reviewed Scientific Papers, Official Reports, Books and Book Chapters on MCS." MCS Referral & Resources. http://mcsrr.org/resources/bibliography.

_____. "Biomarkers of MCS and Muses Syndrome." MCS Referral & Resources. May 11, 2006. www.mcsrr.org/resources/biomarkers.html.

_____. "Recognition of MCS As a Legitimate Disease and Disability." MCS Referral & Resources, October 23, 2006. www.mcsrr.org/factsheets/mcsrecog.html.

_____. "Recognition of Multiple Chemical Sensitivity." August 15, 1998. MCS Referral & Resources. www.mcsrr.org/factsheets/MCSrecogn.pdf.

European Commission. "What is Reach?" 2007. http://ec.europa.eu/environment/chemicals/reach/reach_intro.htm.

Fasey, Andrew, "REACH Is Here: The Politics Are Over, Now the Hard Work Starts." March 2007. http://www.chemicalspolicy.org/downloads/REACHisHere220307.pdf.

Fujimaki H., Sasaki, F. "Effect of Prolonged Exposure to Low Concentrations of Formaldehyde on the Corticotropin Releasing Hormone Neurons in the Hypothalamus and Adrenocorticotropic Hormone Cells in the Pituitary Gland in Female Mice." *Brain Research* July 2, 2004; 1013(1):10716. www.ncbi.nlm.nih.gov/pubmed/15196973?dopt=AbstractPlus.

Genser, Julie. "Safer Construction Tips for the Environmentally Sensitive." Planet Thrive. 2007. http://www.planetthrive.com/members/PDFs/Safer%20Construction%20Tips%20read%20only.pdf.

Gershon, David, and Gail Straub. *Empowerment: The Art of Creating Your Life As You Want It.* West Hurley, N.Y.: High Point Press, 1989.

Gonzales, Claire. "Example MCS Disability EEOC Guidance Letter." U.S. Equal Employment Opportunity Commission. July 24, 1996. www.jan.wvu.edu/letters/EEOC Letter_MCS_Disability_July_96.doc.

Hay, Louise L. *You Can Heal Your Life.* West Carlsbad, Calif.: Hay House, 1999.

Heuser, G., Axelrod, P., and Heuser, S. "Defining Chemical Injury: A Diagnostic Protocol and Profile of Chemically Injured Civilians, Industrial Workers and Gulf War." *International Perspectives in Public*

Health, Fall 2000; 13:1–16. www.iicph.org/docs/ipph_Defining_Chemical_Injury.htm.

Hooper, Malcolm. "Engaging with Multiple Chemical Sensitivity (MCS)." http://www.satori-5.co.uk/word_articles/mcs/engaging_with_mcs.html.

The Interagency Workgroup on Multiple Chemical Sensitivity. "A report on Multiple Chemical Sensitivity (MCS)." August 24, 1998. http://www.health.gov/environment/mcs.

Johnson, Alison. *Casualties of Progress: Personal Histories from the Chemically Sensitive.* Brunswick, Me.: MCS Information Exchange, 2000.

Lee, John R. "Environmental Illness: Could Chemical Overload Be the Cause of Your Illness?" Interview with William J. Rea, M.D., Huntington Beach, Calif. http://www.johnleemd.com/store/env_illness.html.

McCampbell, Ann. "Multiple Chemical Sensitivities under Siege." Townsend Letter for Doctors and Patients, Issue 210, January 2001. www.mindfully.org/Health/MCS-Under-Siege.htm.

McKeown-Eyssen, G., et al. "Case-Control Study of Genotypes in Multiple Chemical Sensitivity: CYP2D6, NAT1, NAT2, PON1, PON2, and MTHFR." *International Journal of Epidemiology.* IJE Advance Access published online on July 15, 2004. http://ije.oxfordjournals.org/cgi/reprint/dyh251v1.

McVicker, Marilyn. *Sauna Detoxification Therapy: A Guide for the Chemically Sensitive.* Jefferson, N.C.: McFarland, 1997.

Meggs, William J. "Hypothesis for the Induction and Propagation of Chemical Sensitivity Based on Biopsy Studies." *Environmental Health Perspectives,* March 1997; 105 (suppl. 2):473–478. www.ehponline.org/members/1997/Suppl-2/meggs-full.html.

Miller, Claudia S. "Toxicant-induced Loss of Tolerance: An Emerging Theory of Disease?" *Environmental Health Perspectives,* March 1997; 105(suppl. 2). www.herc.org/news/ehp/miller.html.

_____, and Ashford, Nicholas A. *Chemical Exposures: Low Levels and High Stakes.* New York: John Wiley & Sons, 1998.

Nethercott J.R., Davidoff L.L., Curbow B., Abbey H. "Multiple Chemical Sensitivities Syndrome: Toward a Working Case Definition." *Archives of Environmental Health* 1993; 48:19–26. www.ncbi.nlm.nih.gov/pubmed/8452395?dopt=Abstract.

"No Safe Haven: People with Multiple Chemical Sensitivity Are Becoming the New Homeless." *E, The Environmental Magazine,* Volume IX, Number 5, September/October 1998. http://www.emagazine.com/view/?1003.

Pall, Martin. "Elevated Nitric Oxide/Peroxynitrite Theory of Multiple Chemical Sensitivity: Central Role of N-Methyl-d-Aspartate Receptors in the Sensitivity Mechanism." *Environmental Health Perspectives* September 2003; 111(12):1461–1464. www.ehponline.org/members/2003/5935/5935.html.

Radetsky, Peter. *Allergic to the Twentieth Century.* Boston: Little, Brown, 1997.

Rajhathy, Judit. *Free to Fly: A Journey toward Wellness.* Halifax, N.S.: New World Publishing, 1999.

Rapp, Doris J. *Our Toxic World: A Wake-Up Call.* Buffalo, N.Y.: Environmental Research Foundation, 2004.

Rea, William J. *Chemical Sensitivity: Tools for Diagnosis and Methods of Treatment Volume IV.* Boca Raton, Fla.: CRC Press, 1997.

_____. "Environmentally Triggered Disorders." *Sandorama* IV, 1982, pp. 27–31. www.aehf.com/articles/A19.htm.

Reed Gibson, Pamela, Elms, Amy Nicole-Marie and Ruding, Lisa Ann. "Perceived Treatment Efficacy for Conventional and Alternative Therapies Reported by Persons with Multiple Chemical Sensitivity." *Environmental Health Perspectives* September 2003; 111(12). http://www.ehponline.org/members/2003/5936/5936.html.

Ridings, Janine. *Comfort in the Storm: Devotions for the Chemically Sensitive.* Enumclaw, Wa.: Pleasant Word, 2004.

Robbins, Anthony. *Unlimited Power: The New Science of Personal Achievement.* New York: Free Press, 1997.

Rogers, Sherry A. *Chemical Sensitivity, Environmental Diseases and Pollutants: How*

They Hurt Us, How to Deal with Them. New Canaan, Conn.: Keats Publishing, 1995.

_____. *Detoxify or Die.* Sarasota, Fla.: Sand Key Company, 2002.

Ross, G.H., Rea, W.J., Johnson, A.R., Hickey, D.C., Simon, T.R. "Neurotoxicity in Single Photon Emission Computed Tomography Brain Scans of Patients Reporting Chemical Sensitivities." *Toxicology and Industrial Health* April–June 1999; 15(3–4):415–420. www.ncbi.nlm.nih.gov/pubmed/10416294?dopt=AbstractPlus.

Saito, M., et al. "Symptom Profile of Multiple Chemical Sensitivity in Actual Life," *Psychosomatic Medicine* March–April 2005; 67(2):318–325. www.ncbi.nlm.nih.gov/pubmed/15784800?dopt=Abstract.

Salvador, Lourdes. "Position Statement: Multiple Chemical Sensitivity." 2007. MCS America. http://mcs-america.org/MCSPositionStatement.pdf.

Sari, D.K., et al. "A Cross-Sectional Study of Self-Reported Chemical-Related Sensitivity Is Associated with Gene Variants of Drug-Metabolizing Enzymes." *Environmental Health* February 10, 2007; 6:6. www.ncbi.nlm.nih.gov/pubmed/17291352?dopt=Abstract.

Sears, Margaret E. "The Medical Perspective on Environmental Sensitivities." May 2007. Canadian Human Rights Commission. www.chrc-ccdp.ca/pdf/envsensitivity_en.pdf.

Sorg, B.A., et al. "Exposure to Repeated Low-Level Formaldehyde in Rats Increases Basal Corticosterone Levels and Enhances the Corticosterone Response to Subsequent Formaldehyde." *Brain Research* April 20, 2001; 898(2):31420. www.ncbi.nlm.nih.gov/pubmed/11306018?dopt=AbstractPlus.

Spivey, Angela. "Genes and Sensitivity." *Environmental Health Perspectives* March 2005; 113:3. http://www.ehponline.org/docs/2005/113-3/forum.html#gene.

Sullivan Restivo, Gail. "Multiple Chemical Sensitivities: Facts, Fiction, Disability and the Law." 2006. 'Lectric Law Library. www.lectlaw.com/filesh/csl01.htm.

The U.S. Department of Education. "Multiple Chemical Sensitivity." Information Memorandum RSA-IM-02-04, November 5, 2001. www.ed.gov/policy/speced/guid/rsa/im/2002/im-02-04.pdf.

Valkenburg-Walsteijn, Els. *Het ABC van Reiki.* Schors, Amsterdam, 2005. www.het-abc-van-reiki.nl/en.

Wilson, Carole W. "MCS Disorder and Environmental Illness As Handicaps." March 5, 1992. The U.S. Department of Housing and Urban Development. www.hud.gov/offices/adm/hudclips/lops/GME-0009LOPS.pdf.

World Health Organization. "Almost a Quarter of All Disease Caused by Environmental Exposure." June 2006. http://www.who.int/mediacentre/news/releases/2006/pr32/en/index.html.

World Health Organization Sustainable Development and Healthy Environments. "International Statistical Classification of Diseases and Related Health Problems (ICD-10) in Occupational Health." WHO/SDE/OEH/99-11. 1999. www.who.int/occupational_health/publications/en/oehicd10.pdf.

Zwillinger, Rhonda. *The Dispossessed — Living with Multiple Chemical Sensitivities.* Paulden, Ariz.: The Dispossessed Project, 1998.

Interviews

Abod, Susan (*entry 98*), Email, January 15, 2007

Annelies (*entry 114*), Email, October 29, 2006

Anonymous (entry 108), Email, December 5, 2006

Anonymous (*entry 112*), Email, October 24, 2006

Anonymous (*entry 115*), Email, January 17, 2007

Anonymous (*entry 118*), Email, November 15, 2006

Anonymous (*entry 122*), Email, January 22, 2007

BubbleGirl, Season (*entry 101*), December 23, 2006

Buckland, Diana (*entry 99*), Email December 7, 2006

Genser, Julie (*entry 97*), Email, December 24, 2006

Guthrie, Graham (*entry 100*), Email, December 26, 2006

Johnson, Alison (*entry 95*), Email, December 26, 2006

Jolanda (*entry 107*), Email, October 24, 2006

Kongevang, Helle (*entry 102*), Email, December 28, 2006

Margot (*entry 110*), Email, January 5, 2007

Marianne (*entry 113*), Email, October 23, 2006

McHendry, Gordon D. (*entry 105*), Email, December 20, 2006

McNeill, Moon (*entry 103*), Email, December 07, 2006

Müller, Silvia (*entry 104*), Email and Telephone, December 6, 2006

Nieuwkoop, Dick van (*entry 116*), Email, January 5, 2007

Prasing, Dick (*entry 111*), Email, January 23, 2007

Ruijter, Mirjam (*entry 117*), Email, October 24, 2006

Salvador, Lourdes (*entry 94*), Email, December 6, 2006

Schifferle, Christian (*entry 106*), Email, December 25, 2006

Schneider, Willem (*entry 119*), Email, November 16, 2006

Slenders, Julia (*entry 109*), Telephone and Fax, January 15, 2007

Terpstra, Annie (*entry 120*), Email, January 8, 2007

Theo (*entry 121*), Email, December 16, 2006

Troiano, Peggy (*entry 96*), Email, December 12, 2006

Index

Numbers are to entry numbers, not pages.